JAMES G. MARKS, JR., M.D.

OCCUPATIONAL SKIN DISORDERS

OCCUPATIONAL SKIN DISORDERS

Daniel J. Hogan, M.D.
Chief of Dermatology
Bay Pines VA Medical Center
Bay Pines, Florida

    and

Professor, Department of Medicine
  (Dermatology and Cutaneous Surgery)
Professor, Department of Pediatrics
  (Dermatology and Cutaneous Surgery)
College of Medicine
University of South Florida
Professor of Environmental and Occupational Health
Department of Public Health
University of South Florida
Tampa, Florida

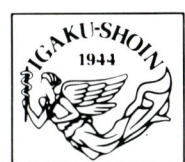

IGAKU-SHOIN New York • Tokyo

Published and distributed by

IGAKU-SHOIN Medical Publishers, Inc.
One Madison Avenue, New York, New York 10010

IGAKU-SHOIN Ltd.,
5-24-3 Hongo, Bunkyo-ku, Tokyo 113-91.

Copyright © 1994 by IGAKU-SHOIN Medical Publishers, Inc.
All rights reserved. No part of this book may be translated or reproduced in any form by print, photo-print, microfilm or any other means without written permission from the publisher.

Library of Congress Cataloging-in-Publication Data

Occupational skin disorders / [edited by] Daniel J. Hogan.
    p. cm.
  Includes bibliographical references and index.
  1. Occupational dermatitis. I. Hogan, Daniel J., M.D.
  [DNLM: 1. Dermatitis, Occupational—diagnosis. 2. Dermatitis, Occupational—therapy. WR 600 01555 1994]
RL241.0274 1994
616.5'1—dc20
DNLM/DLC
for Library of Congress   94-1678
                                                    CIP

ISBN: 0-89640-248-7 (New York)
ISBN: 4-260-14248-8 (Tokyo)

Printed and bound in the U.S.A.

10 9 8 7 6 5 4 3 2 1

Preface

An occupational skin disease is one wholly or partially due to the patient's occupation. Individuals, particularly men, usually identify themselves by the type of work they do. For most people, work is a vital psychological part of their lives. In addition to the adverse psychological effects of being off work, most individuals who stop working or change occupations because of occupational dermatoses suffer a substantial financial loss that is permanent. This is especially true for older workers whose opportunities for alternate employment are significantly limited. The longer a worker is off work, the less likely the worker is to ever to return to work. Prompt and thorough evaluation at an early stage has important benefits for the worker and patient and is the impetus for this text.

Occupational contact dermatitis is the most common occupational dermatosis and the major topic of this text. Drs. Shenefelt, Goldner, and Jackson expertly review allergic contact dermatitis and irritant contact dermatitis in the first two chapters. Dermatologists are the physicians best qualified to diagnose and manage occupational dermatoses and Dr. Fransway authoritatively emphasizes the importance of accurate diagnosis in Chapter 3. Drs. Gallant, Sherertz, and Daily provide a wealth of practical advice on basic patch testing for the occupational dermatologist in Chapters 4, 5, and 6. Drs. Tanglertsampan and Maibach provide a succinct update on contact urticaria in Chapter 7. Other skin diseases, including some that are frequently seen by all dermatologists, may be of occupational origin and are reviewed in Chapter 8 by Drs. Ruxin and Taylor. Treatment is an infrequently discussed topic in occupational dermatology; Dr. Fowler gives practical guidance on treatment options in Chapter 9.

Most physicians receive very little training in occupational medicine. Most dermatologists receive minimal training in occupational dermatology during their dermatologic residencies. These factors contribute to the lack of interest of many dermatologists in occupational dermatology. Occupational skin disorders are noteworthy for the importance of obtaining a detailed and complete history. Virtually all dermatologists are handicapped by their isolation from the patient's workplace. Dermatologists received fragmented information about working conditions and workplace exposures. Accurate diagnosis and dermatologic management require detailed information about both the job and the workplace. Dr. Dannaker provides an excellent introduction to this complex arena in Chapter 10.

Another central problem in occupational dermatology is the artificial distinction between work-related and nonwork-related dermatologic disorders. From a medical perspective there is no need to maintain a separate system of care and compensation for work-related dermatologic problems. Dermatologic expertise and knowledge are necessary to evaluate and diagnose appropriately an occupational dermatosis. Quibbling over the contribution of the workplace to the patient's dermatitis is often a legal rather than a medical issue with financial implications for all concerned. Mr. Swanson presents the essential practical legal information on workers' compensation in Chapter 11.

We believe that this text provides the basic information required by the clinical dermatologist who is the physician best qualified to manage occupational and nonoccupational dermatoses. Once an accurate diagnosis is made, the investigative and management techniques outlined by the experts in this text provide practical guidance to work-related dermatoses. We hope this text will assist clinical dermatologists in this complex yet vital part of dermatology.

Daniel J. Hogan, M.D.

Contributors

Arthur D. Daily, M.D.
Clinical Associate Professor of Medicine
Brown University
Providence, Rhode Island
Assistant Clinical Professor of Dermatology
Boston University
Boston, Massachusetts

Christopher J. Dannaker, M.D.
Assistant Professor
Department of Dermatology
University of California, San Francisco
San Francisco, California

Joseph F. Fowler, Jr., M.D.
Associate Clinical Professor
Director of Occupational Dermatology and Patch Test Clinic
Division of Dermatology
University of Louisville
Louisville, Kentucky

Anthony F. Fransway, M.D.
Assistant Clinical Professor
Department of Dermatology
University of South Florida
Tampa, Florida

Christopher J. Gallant, M.D., M.Sc., F.R.C.P.C.
Assistant Professor
Department of Medicine
Division of Dermatology
Dalhousie University
Halifax, Nova Scotia
Canada

Ronald Goldner, M.D., F.A.C.P.
Clinical Associate Professor
Department of Dermatology
University of Maryland
Baltimore, Maryland

Edward M. Jackson, Ph.D.
President, Jackson Research Associates, Inc.
Cincinnati, Ohio
Associate Adjunct Professor of Pharmaceutics
University of Maryland School of Pharmacy
Baltimore, Maryland
Clinical Assistant Professor
Department of Dermatology
University of Cincinnati School of Medicine
Cincinnati, Ohio

Howard I. Maibach, M.D.
Professor, Department of Dermatology
University of California School of Medicine
San Francisco, California

Tamra A. Ruxin, M.D.
Senior Resident
Department of Dermatology
The Cleveland Clinic Foundation
Cleveland, Ohio

Philip D. Shenefelt, M.D., M.S.
Department of Internal Medicine
Division of Dermatology and Cutaneous Surgery
College of Medicine
University of South Florida
Tampa, Florida

Elizabeth F. Sherertz, M.D.
Department of Dermatology
Wake Forest University Medical Center
Medical Center Boulevard
Winston-Salem, North Carolina

Douglas A. Swanson, J.D.
Royce, Swanson, Thomas & Coon
Attorneys at Law
Portland, Oregon

Chuchai Tanglertsampan, M.D.
Department of Dermatology
University of California School of Medicine
San Francisco, California

James S. Taylor, M.D.
Head, Section of Industrial Dermatology
Department of Dermatology
The Cleveland Clinic Foundation
Cleveland, Ohio

Dedicated to Lory, Gregory, and Matthew

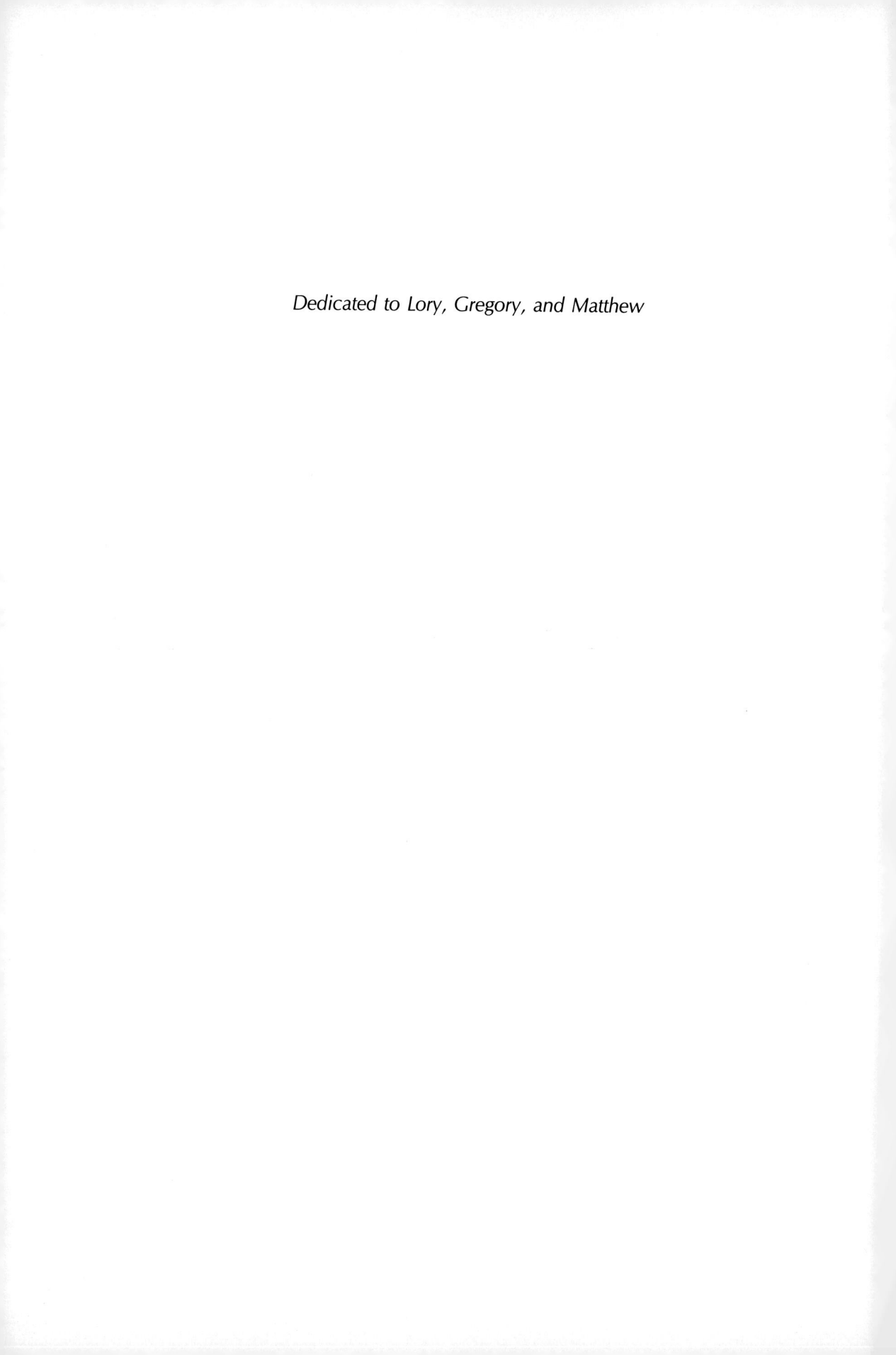

Contents

Chapter 1	**Clinical Aspects of Occupational Allergic Contact Dermatitis** 1 Philip D. Shenefelt	
Chapter 2	**Irritant Contact Dermatitis** 13 Ronald Goldner Edward M. Jackson	
Chapter 3	**The Differential Diagnosis of Occupational Dermatoses** 24 Anthony F. Fransway	
Chapter 4	**Patch Testing a Century Later** 41 Christopher J. Gallant	
Chapter 5	**Patch Testing Using Standard Screening Sets for Cases of Occupational Dermatitis** 54 Elizabeth F. Sherertz	
Chapter 6	**Patch Testing to Allergens Not Found in the Standard Trays** 70 Arthur D. Daily	
Chapter 7	**Contact Urticaria** 81 Chuchai Tanglertsampan Howard I. Maibach	
Chapter 8	**Other Occupational Dermatoses: Acne, Pigmentary Disorders, Skin Cancer, Infection, Reactions to Temperature and Humidity, Scleroderma, and Nail Changes** 89 Tamra A. Ruxin James S. Taylor	

Chapter 9   Treatment of Occupational Dermatitis   104
            Joseph F. Fowler, Jr.

Chapter 10 Nondermatologic Aspects of Occupational
            Dermatology   112
            Christopher J. Dannaker

Chapter 11 Dealing with Workers' Compensation Boards   129
            Douglas A. Swanson

Appendix 1 North American Contact Dermatitis Group Standard
            Allergens   141
            True Test   142
            Commercial Patch Test Trays Available from
            Chemotechnique and Hermal/Trolab   143

Appendix 2 Distributors of Chemical Resistance Charts for Work
            and General Gloves   158

Appendix 3 Distributors of Hypoallergic Gloves and Products   159

Appendix 4 Common Latex Examination Gloves and Their
            Associated Antigens   160

Appendix 5 Societies and Their Journals for Dermatologists
            Interested in Contact Dermatitis and Occupational
            Dermatoses   163

Index   165

Color Plates

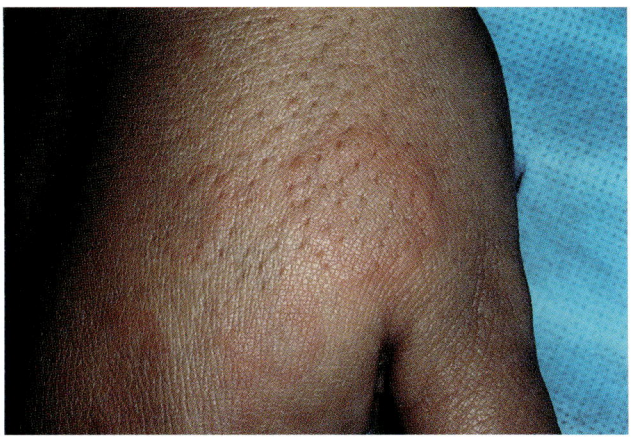

Plate 1-1. Contact urticaria on the dorsum of the right hand due to immediate contact sensitivity to a latex glove in a nurse's aide.

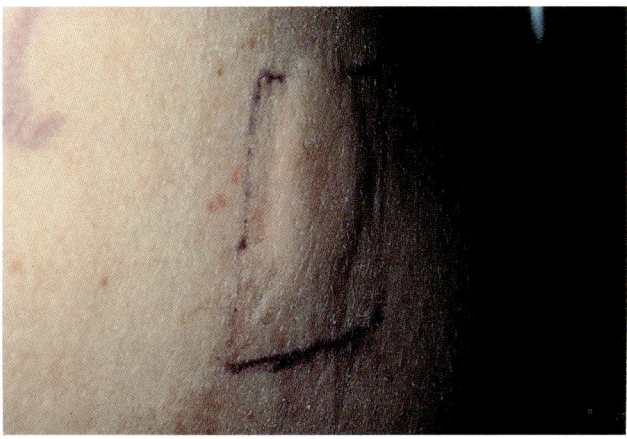

Plate 1-2. Contact urticaria reproduced on the back of the nurse's aide by application of a piece of latex glove.

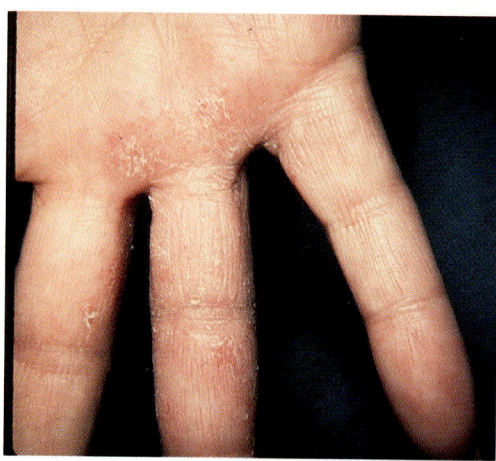

Plate 1-3. Dyshidrosis on the right palm. Note the "apron" involvement on the palm at the base of the digit.

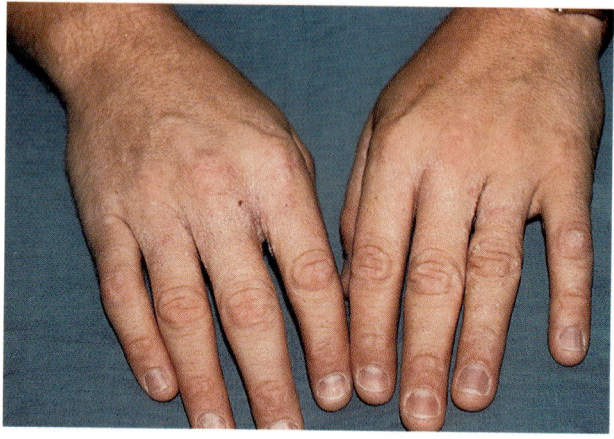

Plate 1-4. Irritant contact dermatitis in fingerwebs of hands due to repeated exposure to soapy solutions.

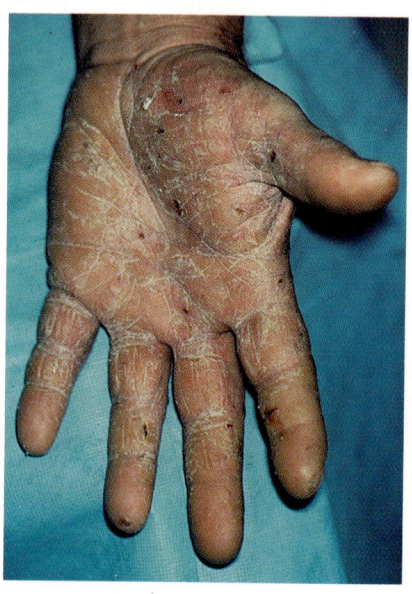

Plate 1-5. Irritant contact dermatitis to paint thinner and hand cleansers in a cabinet maker.

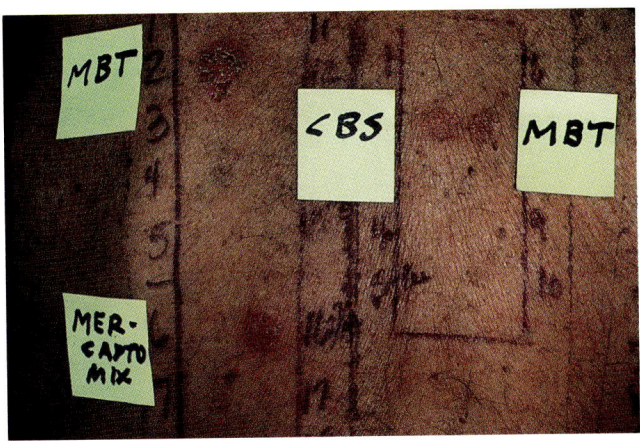

Plate 1-6. Positive patch tests to rubber chemicals on the back of the automobile mechanic.

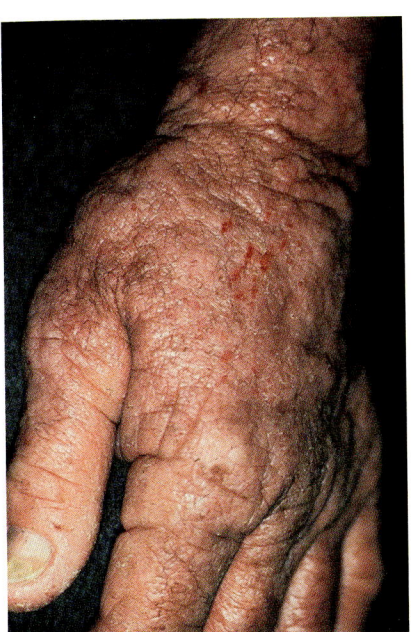 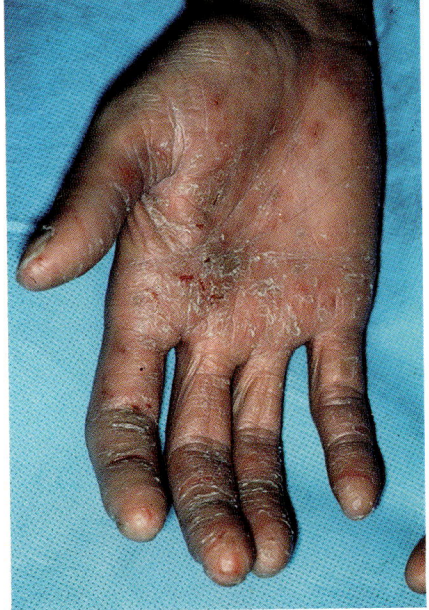

Plate 1-7. Chronic lichenified allergic contact dermatitis in an automobile mechanic.

Plate 1-8. Allergic contact dermatitis involving the entire right hand in a nurse sensitive to latex gloves.

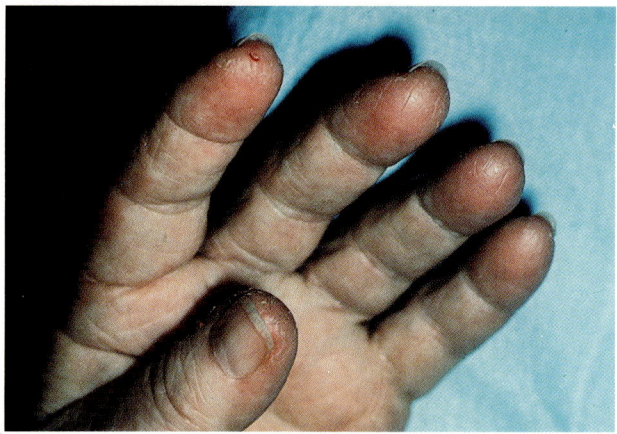

Plate 1-9. Dry, fissured allergic contact dermatitis of the fingertips in an office worker shown by patch testing to be sensitive to paraphenylenediamine and nickel.

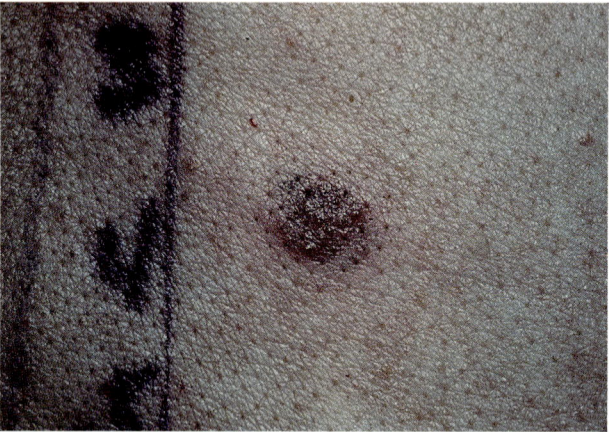

Plate 1-10. Positive patch test to paraphenylenediamine in the office worker. Note the dark stain produced by the polymerized paraphenylenediamine.

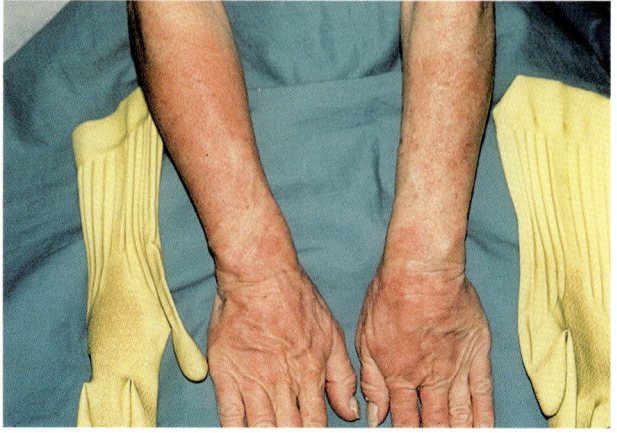

Plate 1-11. Allergic contact allergy to protective rubber gloves. Note the sharp cutoff at the glove line.

1

Clinical Aspects of Occupational Allergic Contact Dermatitis

Philip D. Shenefelt

Allergic contact dermatitis is a common and often costly cause of worker disability. Over 3000 chemicals are recognized as potential contact allergens.[1] Many of these are found in the workplace under conditions conducive to heavy and repeated exposure. Once sensitized, the worker often experiences a number of sick days due to the dermatitis.[2] Cross-sensitization to compounds with a similar molecular configuration may also occur. Discovering the cause of the dermatitis permits proper management of the patient. Changing the work methods to avoid contact with the sensitizer or, in exceptional cases, changing jobs is required to facilitate resolution of the dermatitis. Even after contact ceases, complete resolution of the dermatitis is not guaranteed.[3]

Preparing the mind greatly facilitates making a correct diagnosis. Knowing the patterns of presentation and the types of potential irritants and allergens in the workplace helps the physician to choose appropriate tests and treatments. For example, irritant contact dermatitis is far more common in the workplace than is allergic contact dermatitis. However, many of the relatively intractable cases seen by dermatologists turn out to be allergic contact dermatitis, since only small exposures at intervals of a week or two are sufficient to perpetuate this condition. The criteria for differentiating irritant from allergic contact dermatitis are discussed below.

The process of diagnosing occupationally related allergic contact dermatitis contains a number of pitfalls for the unwary. The following questions, taken in sequence, can help to reduce diagnostic errors:

1. Is it really dermatitis?
2. Is the dermatitis really due to exogenous contact?
3. Is the contact dermatitis really allergic?
4. Is the allergic contact dermatitis really related to the patient's occupation?

These questions will now be discussed in detail.

IS IT REALLY DERMATITIS?

Dermatitis is a superficial inflammatory process involving the epidermis and upper dermis. The process can have an exogenous or endogenous cause. It can be acute, with marked erythema and vesiculation; subacute, with erythema and scaling or fissuring; or chronic, with lichenification.

The differential diagnosis of acute dermatitis includes vesiculobullous disorders such as bullous impetigo, eczema herpeticum, bullous pemphigoid, bullous drug eruption, and bullous erythema multiforme. It also includes conditions producing erythema such as erysipelas, toxic erythema, viral exanthem, drug eruption, and scarlatina. For subacute dermatitis, the differential diagnosis includes erythematous and/or scaly disorders such as eczematous polymorphous light eruption, intertrigo, familial benign chronic pemphigus (Hailey-Hailey disease), tinea, erythrasma, pemphigus foliaceous, psoriasis, parapsoriasis, pityriasis rubra pilaris, Bowen's disease, Paget's disease, and early mycosis fungoides. The differential diagnosis of chronic dermatitis includes hyperkeratotic processes such as lichen simplex chronicus, Norwegian scabies, and psoriasis.[4] The differential diagnosis of occupational dermatoses is discussed in detail in chapter 3.

Differentiating among these disease processes must be done by a careful history and physical examination. In many cases, differentiation may be made on clinical grounds alone, but in other, less clear-cut cases, appropriate laboratory tests and skin biopsies, where necessary, are warranted.

Immediate hypersensitivity contact urticaria must also be differentiated from delayed hypersensitivity allergic contact dermatitis. Contact urticaria may occur on either a pharmacologic or an allergic basis. The most common nonallergic contact urticant is cinnamic aldehyde. Stinging, itching, erythema, or whealing usually occurs within a few minutes to 30 min after exposure.[5] The protein in latex rubber is becoming one of the most common allergic contact urticants.[6] (Plates 1-1 and 1-2). Several anaphylactic deaths have recently been reported from immediate contact sensitivity to latex rubber. Contact urticaria is reviewed in detail in chapter 7.

IS IT EXOGENOUS CONTACT DERMATITIS?

Once the diagnosis of dermatitis has been established, the cause of the dermatitis should be sought. Dermatitis can be due to exogenous contact, endogenous factors, or a combination of both.[7] Common endogenous dermatitides include seborrheic dermatitis, atopic dermatitis, stasis dermatitis, dyshidrosis (Plate 1-3), and nummular dermatitis. In atopic dermatitis, irritant contact dermatitis from detergents or solvents may be an exacerbating factor. However, chronic dermatidities such as atopic dermatitis or stasis dermatitis can be complicated by the development of an allergic contact dermatitis to an ingredient in one of the topical treatments used. When an endogenous dermatitis fails to improve with treatment, patch testing should be considered to rule out superimposed allergic contact dermatitis. Increasingly, contact allergy to corticosteroids is being recognized.[8]

Contact dermatitis typically occurs in sites exposed to the offending agent, although the hands can transfer it to other sites such as the face or genitalia. A sharp demarcation of the dermatitis favors an exogenous contact source. Although usually confluent, contact dermatitis may occasionally be patchy or even follicular in distribution.

IS IT ALLERGIC CONTACT DERMATITIS?

Differentiation of allergic from irritant contact dermatitis may be difficult on clinical grounds. Irritant contact dermatitis involves skin damage without immune-mediated immediate or delayed hypersensitivity. A history of exposure is often helpful. With a strong irritant, the patient can usually relate the contact with the dermatitis. However, with weaker irritants such as water, detergents, mild solvents, and waterless hand cleansers, the repetitive mild injury with its cumulative effect may not be so readily apparent.

Irritant contact dermatitis may present with one of several clinical patterns. The dermatitis may be dry and fissured without erythema. This pattern is often produced by dusty, dirty environments. The dermatitis may be dry, fissured, and erythematous (Plates 1-4 and 1-5). Often wet work produces this pattern. The dermatitis may be vesicular, dry, and fissured, with or without erythema. This pattern may simulate dyshidrosis.

The diagnostic criteria for irritant contact dermatitis developed by Rietschel[9] may be helpful in separating irritant from allergic contact dermatitis. Subjective major criteria for irritant contact dermatitis are onset of symptoms within minutes to hours of exposure and primarily pain, burning, stinging, or discomfort rather than itching. Subjective minor criteria are onset of dermatitis within 2 weeks of exposure and many people in the environment similarly affected. Objective major criteria are erythema, hyperkeratosis, or fissuring predominating over vesicles; a glazed, parched, or scalded appearance; relatively rapid healing following cessation of exposure; and negative patch tests to relevant allergens. Objective minor criteria include sharp circumscription of the dermatitis, evidence of gravitational flow such as dripping, lack of progressive spreading of the dermatitis, and closely juxtaposed patches of vesicles, erythema, erosions, and fissures suggesting large differences in skin damage, with small changes in concentration or contact time (see Table 2-5, p. 19).

With allergic contact dermatitis, the patient may associate an exposure followed by dermatitis several days to several weeks later. The patient may have been exposed for weeks, months, or years before becoming allergic to a chemical. Sometimes the patient's idea of which exposure is leading to the dermatitis is correct, but often it is not. If the relationship between exposure and dermatitis is clear-cut, based on the history, simple avoidance may solve the problem. If not, patch testing is indicated once the dermatitis is sufficiently subdued to minimize the angry back syndrome.[10] Patch testing will help to differentiate between irritant and allergic contact dermatitis and will often identify the offending antigen in the case of allergic contact dermatitis[11,12] (Plate 1-6). Vesicles may predominate in acute allergic contact dermatitis. Chronic allergic contact dermatitis tends to assume a more dry, lichenified, or fissured appearance (Plate 1-7). Usually a patient with allergic contact dermatitis complains of itching rather than burning.

When suggested by the distribution in light-exposed areas, phototoxic or photoallergic contact reactions must also be considered.[13] Usually there is sparing of shaded areas with photodermatitis. Photopatch testing is indicated in cases of suspected photoallergic contact dermatitis.

IS IT RELATED TO THE PATIENT'S OCCUPATION?

Once a skin eruption has been identified as allergic contact dermatitis, it is necessary to determine whether it is related to the patient's occupation. If the only exposure of the patient to the allergen is in the workplace, this determination is simple. However, exposure to many common allergens may occur outside of the workplace. Examples are nickel, rubber chemicals, ingredients in topical lotions, antibiotics, and other topical medications, cosmetic and toiletry products, fabrics, glues, and sundry other materials with which the patient may come into contact outside of the work setting.

The patient's history, along with Material Safety Data Sheets (MSDSs) for all chemicals to which the patient is exposed, are a starting place for evaluating the chemical exposure in the workplace. However, chemicals present in less than a 1% concentration are not required to be listed on MSDSs, yet these chemicals may be in sufficient concentration to elicit allergic contact dermatitis.[14] The most useful information on the MSDS is often the telephone number of the manufacturer. If the manufacturer is reluctant to disclose whether a particular allergen is present in a product, a telephone call to the Environmental Protection Agency may force the manufacturer to release medically necessary information.

A site visit to the workplace to search for possible sources of a particular allergen for which the patient is patch test positive may be necessary. It is preferable to visit while the production activity in which the patient is involved is going on.

REGIONAL DISTRIBUTION OF IRRITANT AND ALLERGIC CONTACT DERMATITIS

The hands are the most frequently involved area in both irritant and allergic contact dermatitis. In some occupations where exposure is uniform over the whole hand, the dermatitis will usually cover the entire hand (Plate 1-8). In other occupations, such as that of florist, only the thumb and forefinger may be involved (Plates 1-9 and 1-10). Allergic contact dermatitis can be patchy, can involve the palms, and can be present in individuals with another preexisting dermatosis.[13]

The forearms and distal arms may be involved as an extension of the hands, or may be involved while the glove-protected hands remain uninvolved. Again, the dermatitis may be patchy or confluent. A sharp cutoff of the dermatitis at the sleeve line or glove line (Plate 1-11) is a good indicator that an exogenous dermatitis is present.

The face and neck may be exposed to sprays or dust, but more commonly the hands transfer chemicals to these areas. The skin on the face, particularly the eyelids, absorbs chemicals more readily than do the hands.

The genitals also absorb chemicals readily. Transfer of chemicals from the hands to this area is common in men. Irritant or allergic contact dermatitis may result.

Clothed areas may develop irritant or allergic contact dermatitis from materials in the clothing itself, from laundering agents, or from chemicals that have soaked through the clothing.

Generalized dermatitis may indicate extensive exposure or may result from autoeczematization. Allergic contact dermatitis has a greater tendency to spread than does irritant contact dermatitis.

OCCUPATIONAL GROUPS AND IRRITANT CONTACT DERMATITIS

Exposure to contact irritants is frequent in many occupations. Below are listed the common types of irritants (see Table 1-1, and also Table 2-2, p. 14). Occupational groups in whom irritant skin reactions are likely to occur include agricultural workers, artists, bakers, barbers and hairdressers, bartenders, bathing attendants, bookbinders, building trades workers, butchers, canners, cooks and food preparers, carpenters and woodworkers, chemical and pharmaceutical workers, cleaners, coal and other miners, dental and health care workers, dyers, electricians and electronics workers and repairers, fishermen, florists, gardeners and plant growers, foundry workers, homemakers, jewelers, laundry workers, mechanics, metal platers, metal workers, office workers, painters, photograph developers, plastics workers, plumbers, printers, roofers, rubber workers, shoemakers, tanners, textile workers, veterinarians, and welders (modified from Bruze and Emmett[15]).

Water is a mild irritant. Repetitive, frequent exposures to water remove

TABLE 1-1 Common Contact Irritants

Water
Cleansers and detergents
Organic solvents
Oils and lubricants
Acids
Alkalis
Oxidizing agents and bleaches
Reducing agents
Plants and plant products
Animal products

skin lipids, leading to chapping and fissuring. Wet work is an occupational hazard for barbers and hairdressers, bartenders, bathing attendants, butchers, canners, cooks and food preparers, chemical and pharmaceutical workers, cleaners, coal and other miners, dental and health care workers, fishermen, homemakers, laundry workers, plumbers, and tanners.

Cleansers and detergents defat and damage the stratum corneum, leading to chapping, fissuring, and inflammation. Exposed occupational groups include barbers and hairdressers, agricultural workers, artists, bakers, bartenders, bathing attendants, butchers, canners, cooks and food preparers, carpenters and woodworkers, chemical and pharmaceutical workers, cleaners, dental and health care workers, foundry workers, homemakers, laundry workers, mechanics, metal platers, metal workers, painters, plumbers, printers, roofers, textile workers, and veterinarians.

Organic solvents also defat and damage the stratum corneum. Examples of organic solvents include short chain alcohols such as methanol, ethanol, and isopropanol; aromatic hydrocarbons such as benzene and toluene; chlorinated hydrocarbons such as trichloroethylene; and other solvents such as acetone, turpentine, and paint thinner. Occupational groups at risk include artists, bookbinders, carpenters and woodworkers, chemical and pharmaceutical workers, cleaners, dental and health care workers, dyers, laundry workers, mechanics, metal platers, metal workers, painters, photograph developers, plastics workers, printers, roofers, rubber workers, shoemakers, tanners, and textile workers.

Oils and lubricants replace normal lipids in the stratum corneum. Removing them with solvents or cleansers leads to skin irritation. Cutting oils dry the skin. Exposed occupational groups include agricultural workers, coal and other miners, fishermen, foundry workers, mechanics, metal workers, plumbers, and welders.

Acids vary from strong inorganic acids such as sulfuric and hydrochloric to weak organic acids such as acetic. Exposure of the skin to strong acids can cause chemical burns, while weaker acids may cause dryness and fissuring. Occupational exposure occurs in building trades workers, jewelers, mechanics, metal platers, photograph developers, plastics workers, tanners, and welders.

Alkalis saponify skin surface lipids and damage epidermal cells. Strong alkalis such as potassium hydroxide dissolve skin, while weaker alkalis such as wet concrete, lime, and soap result in drying and fissuring. Occupational groups at risk include building trades, coal and other miners, jewelers, metal platers, photograph developers, and tanners.

Oxidizing agents and bleaches such as hydrogen peroxide and benzoyl peroxide directly damage and kill cells. Exposed occupations include bakers, barbers and hairdressers, dyers, laundry workers, photograph developers, plastics workers, tanners, and textile workers.

Reducing agents such as thioglycolates break disulfide bonds in keratins, damaging the barrier to penetration and may also sensitize some individuals. Occupational groups exposed include barbers and hairdressers, dyers, photograph developers, and tanners.

Plants and plant products can produce contact irritation. Examples are onions, spices, pineapple, and citrus fruits. Occupational groups at risk include agricultural workers, bakers, bartenders, canners, cooks and food preparers, florists, gardeners and plant growers, and homemakers.

Animal products such as meat, fish, and shrimp may cause irritation and contact urticaria. Involved occupational groups include agricultural workers, butchers, canners, cooks and food preparers, fishermen, homemakers, and veterinarians.

Other chemical irritants and potential sensitizers may be encountered in specific work settings. Occupational exposure may occur in agricultural workers (fertilizer, pesticides), bathing attendants (chlorine), bookbinders (glues), building trades workers (wood preservatives, glues), carpenters and woodworkers (wood preservatives, glues), chemical and pharmaceutical workers (specific for each workplace), dental and health care workers (disinfectants, adhesives), electricians and electronics workers and repairers (soldering flux, metal cleaners, epoxy), florists and gardeners and plant growers (fertilizers, pesticides), jewelers (soldering fluxes, adhesives), laundry workers (stain removers), office workers (ammonia from treated papers), painters (paint emulsions, paint removers), plastics workers (monomers), plumbers (soldering fluxes, adhesives), printers (acrylates), roofers (tar, pitch, asphalt), rubber workers (talc, zinc stearate), shoemakers (polishes, glues), and tanners (proteolytic enzymes).

Physical irritants causing microtrauma to the skin may also be encountered in specific types of work.[16] Occupational groups at risk include agricultural workers (grain dust), building trades workers (fiberglass insulation), and florists, gardeners, and plant growers (fibrous hairs on plants).

OCCUPATIONAL GROUPS AND ALLERGIC CONTACT DERMATITIS

The standard Hermal (United States) Allergen Patch Test Kit allergens are listed in Table 1-2 (also see Table 5-1, p 56). These allergens along with the occupations in which exposure to the allergens is likely to occur (modified from Adams[17]) are now discussed.

Cinnamic aldehyde is derived from cinnamon. It is present in many fra-

TABLE 1-2 Hermal (United States) Allergen Patch Test Kit

Allergen	Concentration	Vehicle
1. Benzocaine	5%	Petrolatum
2. Mercaptobenzothiazole	1%	Petrolatum
3. Colophony	20%	Petrolatum
4. Paraphenylenediamine	1%	Petrolatum
5. Imidazolidinyl urea	2%	Water
6. Cinnamic aldehyde	1%	Petrolatum
7. Lanolin alcohol	30%	Petrolatum
8. Carba mix	3%	Petrolatum
9. Neomycin sulfate	20%	Petrolatum
10. Thiuram mix	1%	Petrolatum
11. Formaldehyde	1%	Water
12. Ethylenediamine dihydrochloride	1%	Petrolatum
13. Epoxy resin	1%	Petrolatum
14. Quaternium 15	2%	Petrolatum
15. Paratertiary-butylphenol formaldehyde resin	1%	Petrolatum
16. Mercapto mix	1%	Petrolatum
17. Black rubber paraphenylenediamine mix	0.6%	Petrolatum
18. Potassium dichromate	0.25%	Petrolatum
19. Balsam of Peru	25%	Petrolatum
20. Nickel sulfate	2.5%	Petrolatum

grances, flavorings, and bakery goods. In addition to ordinary allergic contact dermatitis, it can produce bullous eruptions and nonimmunologic immediate contact urticaria. Occupational groups affected include bakers, bartenders, bathing attendants, canners, cooks and food preparers, and dental workers.

Paraphenylenediamine is a colorless compound that polymerizes into a black dye used for hair, shoes, fabrics, and printing inks. Patients with paraphenylenediamine allergy may develop a cross-reaction to other para compounds such as benzocaine, para-aminobenzoic acid (PABA) sunscreens, sulfonamides, azo dyes, and others. Contact may occur in several occupational groups, including agricultural workers, artists, barbers and hairdressers, bookbinders, dyers, homemakers, mechanics, painters, printers, rubber workers, shoemakers, tanners, and textile workers.

Epoxy resin is a common adhesive bonding ingredient and is also used in sealants, coatings, and printers' ink. Most two-part glue systems contain epoxy. It is an occupational allergen in artists, bookbinders, building trades workers, carpenters and woodworkers, dental workers, electricians and electronics workers and repairers, homemakers, jewelers, mechanics, painters, plastics workers, plumbers, printers, shoemakers, and textile workers.

Para-tertiary-butylphenol formaldehyde resin is found primarily in leather adhesives and finishes, neoprene adhesives, and weatherstripping. Occupationally exposed workers include agricultural workers, building trades workers, carpenters and woodworkers, electricians and electronics workers and repairers, homemakers, mechanics, office workers, plastics workers, plumbers, shoemakers, tanners, textile workers, and veterinarians.

Imidazolidinyl urea is a formaldehyde-releasing preservative found in hand creams and cosmetics. Occupational exposure occurs in barbers and hairdressers, bathing attendants, homemakers, mechanics, and office workers.

Formaldehyde is a commonly used antimicrobial and industrial chemical. It is found in some shampoos and in nail hardeners, as well as in many industrial cleaners. Occupational exposure may occur in agricultural workers, bakers, barbers and hairdressers, bartenders, bathing attendants, building trades workers, butchers, canners, cooks and food preparers, carpenters and woodworkers, chemical and pharmaceutical workers, cleaners, dental and health care workers, dyers, electricians and electronics workers and repairers, florists, gardeners and plant growers, foundry workers, homemakers, jewelers, laundry workers, mechanics, metal platers, metal workers, office workers, painters, photograph developers, plastics workers, plumbers, printers, roofers, rubber workers, shoemakers, tanners, textile workers, veterinarians, and welders.

Quaternium 15 is a widely used preservative in cosmetics, shampoos, household products, and industry. It is a formaldehyde releaser. The primary occupational groups affected include barbers and hairdressers, bathing attendants, homemakers, mechanics, office workers, and printers.

Balsam of Peru is found in fragrances, medications, and certain woods. It cross-reacts with many fragrance ingredients and is a useful screen for fragrance allergy. The primary occupational groups exposed are barbers and hairdressers, bartenders, bathing attendants, carpenters and woodworkers, dental and health care workers, homemakers, pharmaceutical workers, and veterinarians.

Mercaptobenzothiazole is a rubber accelerator and a frequent sensitizer. It is found in most rubber products. Occupational groups in which sensitization may occur include agricultural workers, barbers and hairdressers, bartenders, building trades workers, butchers, canners, cooks and food preparers, chemical and pharmaceutical workers, cleaners, dental and health care workers, dyers, electricians and electronics workers and repairers, fishermen, florists, gardeners and plant growers, foundry workers, homemakers, laundry workers, mechanics, metal platers, metal workers, office workers, painters, photograph developers, plumbers, printers, roofers, rubber workers, shoemakers, tanners, textile workers, and veterinarians.

Carba mix (1,3-diphenylguanidine, zinc diethyldithiocarbamate, zinc dibutyldithiocarbamate) is a group of rubber accelerators used during the vulcanization process. Certain carbamates are also used as fungicides. Occupational groups in whom sensitization may occur include agricultural workers, artists, bakers, barbers and hairdressers, bartenders, bathing attendants, bookbinders, building trades workers, butchers, canners, cooks and food preparers, carpenters and woodworkers, chemical and pharmaceutical workers, cleaners, coal and other miners, dental and health care workers, dyers, electricians and electronics workers and repairers, fishermen, florists and gardeners and plant growers, homemakers, jewelers, laundry workers, mechanics, metal platers, metal workers, office workers, painters, photograph developers, plastics workers, plumbers, printers, roofers, rubber workers, shoemakers, tanners, textile workers, veterinarians, and welders.

Thiuram mix (tetramethylthiuram disulfide, tetramethylthiuram monosulfide, tetraethylthiuram disulfide, dipentamethylenethiuram disulfide) is a family of rubber accelerators. They are widely used in vulcanization and are frequent sensitizers. Occupational groups with thiuram contact include agricultural workers, artists, bakers, barbers and hairdressers, bartenders, bathing attendants, bookbinders, building trades workers, butchers, canners, cooks and food preparers, carpenters and woodworkers, chemical and pharmaceutical workers, cleaners, coal and other miners, dental and health care workers, dyers, electricians and electronics workers and repairers, fishermen, florists, gardeners and plant growers, homemakers, jewelers, laundry workers, mechanics, metal platers, metal workers, office workers, painters, photograph developers, plastics workers, plumbers, printers, roofers, rubber workers, shoemakers, tanners, textile workers, veterinarians, and welders.

Mercapto mix (*N*-cyclohexyl-2-benzothiazolsulfonamide, 2,2′-benzothiazyl disulfide, 4-morpholinyl-2-benzothiazyl disulfide) is a group of common rubber chemical sensitizers. They serve as accelerators in vulcanization. Occupational groups most affected are agricultural workers, barbers and hairdressers, bartenders, building trades workers, butchers, canners, cooks and food preparers, chemical and pharmaceutical workers, cleaners, dental and health care workers, dyers, electricians and electronics workers and repairers, fishermen, florists, gardeners and plant growers, foundry workers, homemakers, laundry workers, mechanics, metal platers, metal workers, office workers, painters, photograph developers, plumbers, printers, roofers, rubber workers, shoemakers, tanners, textile workers, and veterinarians.

Black rubber mix (*N*-phenyl-*N*′-cyclohexyl-paraphenylenediamine, *N*-isopropyl-*N*′-phenyl-paraphenylenediamine, *N*,*N*′-diphenyl-paraphenylenediamine) causes sensitization primarily in workers involved in tire manufacture. It serves as an antioxidant and is widespread in rubber products including rubber gloves and rubber bands. Those occupational groups mainly at risk of sensitization are agricultural workers, barbers and hairdressers, bartenders, building trades workers, butchers, canners, cooks and food preparers, chemical and pharmaceutical workers, cleaners, dental and health care workers, dyers, electricians, electronics workers and repairers, fishermen, florists and gardeners and plant growers, homemakers, laundry workers, mechanics, metal platers, metal workers, office workers, painters, photograph developers, plumbers, printers, roofers, rubber workers, shoemakers, tanners, textile workers, and veterinarians.

Potassium dichromate is widespread in industry, causing the greatest sensitization problems in cement workers. It can also induce sensitization in artists, building trades workers, carpenters and woodworkers, chemical and pharmaceutical workers, dental and health care workers, dyers, electricians and electronics workers and repairers, jewelers, mechanics, metal platers, metal workers, painters, photograph developers, plumbers, printers, shoemakers, tanners, textile workers, and welders.

Nickel sulfate is a salt of the metal nickel. Nickel is found in most alloys of metal, so exposure to it is widespread but causes proportionately little occupationally induced allergic contact dermatitis. The most common mode of sensitization to nickel is ear piercing, which is not occupationally related. The main workplace exposure is through metal tools in occupational groups such as barbers and hairdressers, building trades workers, dental and health care workers, dyers, electricians, electronics workers and repairers, florists and gardeners and plant growers, foundry workers, homemakers, jewelers, mechanics, metal platers, metal workers, office workers, photograph developers, plumbers, printers, rubber workers, textile workers, and welders.

Lanolin alcohol is a mixture of esters of long chain alcohols and fatty acids extracted from sheep fleece. It is a common ingredient in hand creams. Exposed occupational groups include agricultural workers, bakers, barbers and hairdressers, bathing attendants, building trades workers, chemical and pharmaceutical workers, dental and health care workers, homemakers, laundry workers, mechanics, office workers, printers, shoemakers, tanners, textile workers, and veterinarians.

Benzocaine is a topical anesthetic derived from PABA. It can cross-react with PABA, paraphenylenediamine, sulfonamides, azo dyes, and certain other paracompounds. Occupational exposure may occur in agricultural workers, bathing attendants, dental and health care workers, pharmaceutical workers, and veterinarians.

Colophony or rosin is derived from pine pitch. It is found in wood, sawdust, pine needles, pine cones, cosmetics, adhesives, and solder flux. Occupational exposure may occur in artists, barbers and hairdressers, bookbinders, carpenters and woodworkers, dental workers, electricians and electronics workers and repairers, jewelers, mechanics, metal workers, office workers, painters, plumbers, printers, roofers, rubber workers, shoemakers, tanners, and veterinarians.

Neomycin sulfate is a commonly used topical antibiotic. Occupational exposure occurs in agricultural workers, dental and health care workers, homemakers, pharmaceutical workers and veterinarians, and any worker using triple antibiotic cream (Neosporin) for skin injuries.

Ethylenediamine dihydrochloride was used as a stabilizer in Myclog before it was reformulated. It may still be present in some generic Myclog creams and is present in Tincture of Merthiolate (Lilly). Although it has some industrial uses, few patients become sensitized through industrial contact. Occupations where it may be present include agricultural workers, chemical and pharmaceutical workers, dental and health care workers (ethylenediamine is present in aminophylline), homemakers, painters, photograph developers, rubber workers, textile workers, and veterinarians.

Many other allergens are available in special trays designed to test for common allergens in specific occupations. Examples are dental materials, hairdressing materials, oils and cooling fluids, pesticides, photoallergens, photographic chemicals, plants and woods, plastics and glues, rubber chemicals, shoe chemicals, textile colors and finishes, and vehicles and preservatives (See Appendix 1).[13]

Diagnosing and treating occupational allergic contact dermatitis is a complex and often challenging adventure. Utilizing the above thought patterns and information in an organized approach to occupational dermatitis can produce results that are very rewarding for both physician and patient.

REFERENCES

1. de Groot AC: *Patch Testing.* Amsterdam, Elsevier, 1986.
2. Rycroft RJG: Occupational contact dermatitis. In Rycroft RJG, Menne T, Frosch PJ, et al (eds): *Textbook of Contact Dermatitis.* Berlin, Springer-Verlag, 1992, pp 343–399.
3. Hogan DJ, Dannaker CJ, Maibach HI: Contact dermatitis: Prognosis, risk factors, and rehabilitation. *Semin Dermatol* 9(3):233–246, 1990.
4. Ashton R, Leppard B: *Differential Diagnosis in Dermatology.* Philadelphia, JB Lippincott, 1990.
5. Lahti A, Maibach HI: Immediate contact reactions. In Menne T, Maibach HI (eds): *Exogenous Dermatoses: Environmental Dermatitis.* Boca Raton, FL, CRC Press, 1991, pp 21–35.
6. Sussman GL, Tarlo S, Dolovich J: The spectrum of IgE-mediated responses to latex. *JAMA* 265(21):2844–2847, 1991.
7. Veien NK: Diagnostic procedures for eczema patients. In Menne T, Maibach HI (eds): *Exogenous Dermatoses: Environmental Dermatitis.* Boca Raton, FL, CRC Press, 1991, pp 127–140.
8. Lauerma AI: Contact hypersensitivity to glucocorticosteroids. *Am J Contact Dermatitis* 3(3):112–132, 1992.
9. Rietschel RL: Diagnosing irritant contact dermatitis. In Jackson EM, Goldner R (eds): *Irritant Contact Dermatitis.* New York, Marcel Dekker, 1990, pp 167–171.
10. Bruynzeel DP, Maibach HI: Excited skin syndrome and the hyporeactive state: Current status. In Menne T, Maibach HI (eds): *Exogenous Dermatoses: Environmental Dermatitis.* Boca Raton, FL, CRC Press, 1991, pp 141–150.
11. Fischer T, Maibach HI: Patch testing in allergic contact dermatitis. In Menne T, Maibach HI (eds): *Exogenous Dermatoses: Environmental Dermatitis.* Boca Raton, FL, CRC Press, 1991, pp 85–102.
12. Fisher AA: *Contact Dermatitis,* ed 3. Philadelphia, Lea & Febiger, 1986.
13. Marks JG, DeLeo VA: *Contact and Occupational Dermatology.* St Louis, Mosby Year Book, 1992.
14. Emmett EA: The dermatologist and the right to know. *Dermatol Clin* 6(1):21–26, 1988.
15. Bruze M, Emmett EA: Occupational exposures to irritants. In Jackson EM, Goldner R (eds): *Irritant Contact Dermatitis.* New York, Marcel Dekker, 1990, pp 81–106.
16. Gellin GA: Physical and mechanical causes of occupational dermatoses. In Maibach HI (ed): *Occupational and Industrial Dermatology,* ed 2. Chicago, Year Book, 1987, pp 88–93.
17. Adams RM (ed): *Occupational Skin Disease,* ed 2. Philadelphia, WB Saunders, 1990.

2

Irritant Contact Dermatitis

Ronald Goldner and Edward M. Jackson

SENSITIZATION VERSUS IRRITATION

Irritant contact dermatitis (ICD) is the most frequently made diagnosis of occupationally induced diseases. Yet the diagnosis and treatment of ICD can be one of the most difficult tasks facing the practicing dermatologist. Equally interesting is the continually expanding literature on allergic contact dermatitis (ACD) versus the paucity of literature on ICD. All of us recognize that probing the cellular and molecular events of ACD is much more satisfying than probing the cellular physiology and biochemistry of ICD. But this in itself is not a justification for the lack of clinical and scientific literature on ICD. Finally, clinicians and researchers are at a distinct disadvantage in attempting to find information on ICD.[1]

Why is this? It may well be because irritation tells us something about how we are the same, while sensitization tells us something about how we are different.[2] And writing about differences is much more interesting, but in our opinion less challenging, than writing about sameness.

PATHOPHYSIOLOGY

When the skin is exposed to chemical agents in an occupational setting, several morphologic changes may occur. These changes are produced by contact of the agent with components of the skin. Because of the multitude and frequency of cutaneous exposures to chemicals in the workplace, contact dermatitis is a leading cause of occupational disease.[3]

TABLE 2-1 Bioengineering Techniques to Evaluate Cutaneous Irritation

Technique	Measurement
Laser Doppler velocimetry	Velocity of moving erythrocytes with blood flow
Evaporimeter	Transepidermal Water Loss (TEWL)
Ultrasound	Skin thickness
Impedance, conductance and capacitance	Skin hydration
Colorimeter	Skin coloration

Source: Data from Ref. 6.

The pathophysiology of ICD is best explained by understanding the production of cytokines, adhesion molecules and chemotactic factors from exposed epidermal keratinocytes. The keratinocyte accounts for most cells within the epidermis, and it is certainly not immunologically inert, as was once thought. While the keratinocyte does not routinely express human leukocyte antigen DR (HLA-DR) and is not capable of presenting antigen, it can express other chemical mediators when activated.[4] The activated keratinocyte is capable of producing many mediators of inflammation which allow it to regulate a host of other cells, such as T-lymphocytes, macrophages, mast cells, and vascular endothelial cells.[5]

While ICD is common in the workplace, very few in-depth investigations have been carried out. Bioengineering techniques now make it possible to quantitate minor differences in cutaneous reactivity. Table 2-1 summarizes the most useful techniques available.[6]

TYPES OF IRRITANTS

Any substance that causes direct damage to the skin without prior sensitization can be called a cutaneous irritant. A simple classification of irritants is presented in Table 2-2, but there are wide differences in irritant potential within each of these categories.[7]

Desicants include a number of airborne dusts such as acrylic polymers and food additives. The stratum corneum becomes more brittle and therefore

TABLE 2-2 Types of Irritants

Desicants
Abrasive materials
Organic solvents
Surfactants
Acids and alkalis
Hypertonic solutions
Enzymes

TABLE 2-3 Types of Cosmetic and OTC Drug Products

Decorative cosmetics (facial cosmetics, eye area cosmetics, lip products, and nail care products)

Skin care products (hand and body lotions, facial moisturizers, cleansers, astringents, soap and bath products)

Fragrances (perfumes, colognes, and skin fresheners)

Deodorants and antiperspirants

Shaving products (foams, gels, brushless shaves, aftershave moisturizers, astringents, talcum, styptic sticks, and depilatories)

Oral hygiene products (toothpastes, mouthwashes, and breath fresheners)

Hair products (shampoos, conditioners, hair colorants, curl activators, hair thickeners, sheen products, mousses, styling gels, sprays, bleaches and lighteners, hair straighteners)

Sun protection products (sunscreens, suntan lotions, tan accelerators, self-tanning products)

Feminine hygiene products (douches, feminine deodorants, personal lubricants)

Foot and leg care products (deodorants, depilatories, corn and callus removers)

---

more permeable.[3,8] Abrasive materials include particles of industrial or plant origin. A mechanical irritant dermatitis may result from an accidental exposure. Organic solvents are probably responsible for the majority of cases of occupational irritant dermatitis, possibly by extracting stratum corneum lipids thus compromising the skin's barrier function. Surfactants can also strip stratum corneum lipids, as well as naturally occurring hygroscopic materials. The reasons for the irritation produced by acids and alkalis are not yet well understood. Certainly they can denature proteins, but this does not appear to alter the barrier function. Salt solutions are weak irritants on normal skin but are most irritating when the stratum corneum is damaged. Enzymes such as lipases and proteases produce irritant dermatitis by proteolytic and lipolytic actions.[7,9]

Dermatitis due to consumer products like cosmetics and over-the-counter (OTC) drugs can be part of the spectrum of irritant contact dermatitis. Table 2-3 lists the products patients use and are therefore exposed to. Of these, hair care, shaving, and foot and leg care products are most likely to be implicated in ICD. In some cases, ICD may be due to the actual use of the product, as in repeated shaving. In others, it may be due to the harsh nature of the product itself, such as hair depilatories. But the cumulative effect of subclinical irritation has also been cited as a possible cause.[10] And we cannot dismiss the aggravating effects of certain cosmetic products or their components such as fragrances. It has been suggested that fragrances may in some cases irritate and therefore be possible aggravating factors in contact dermatitis,[11] in addition to being one of the two leading causes of ACD in patients presenting with cosmetic dermatitis.[12,13] Clearly, cosmetics and OTC drugs have the potential to worsen an existing condition and therefore increase the chances for weak allergens to sensitize the patient precisely because the skin is now damaged.

FACTORS IN ICD

Skin irritation is greatly influenced by environmental, host, and penetrability factors. To better understand ICD in the workplace, these factors will be reviewed in detail.

Environmental factors such as cold temperatures and low relative humidity greatly affect the ability of the skin to withstand exposure to irritants. The water content within the stratum corneum is reduced, impairing the barrier function of the skin. Sweating produced by high temperature and elevated humidity may dissolve some irritants and actually increase the skin's exposure to these irritants.[14,15] Environmental factors in ICD vary with the season, as well as with the geographic location.

Host factors are, of course, responsible for differences in ICD. The barrier function of the skin varies significantly with the site and thickness of the skin. As an example, airborne irritant dermatitis is often localized on the face and spares the exposed hands or arms, which are more resistant to cutaneous irritants. There is considerable person-to-person variation in the response to irritants which may be explained by genetic or ethnic differences. Fair skin and blue eyes in Celtic or Scandinavian populations indicates increased sensitivity to irritants.[3,16] Generally, individuals with atopic dermatitis have a higher risk of developing ICD, but anyone with dry skin or xerosis will fare poorly in certain work environments. Sensitivity to irritants seems to increase with age, but irritant reactions tend to persist and be more resistant to therapy in aged skin.[17–20]

Exposure factors and differences in permeability play a significant role in the development of irritant dermatitis. The exposure time and concentration of an irritant have a significant effect on the development of an irritant reaction. Acids and alkalis can readily cause chemical burns, but if the concentration is low and the exposure time is short, only slight erythema may develop. Under occlusion, however, a caustic burn may develop from a chemical that would normally result only in mild dermatitis.[14,21] Chemicals that penetrate defective protective equipment or gloves may produce more severe irritant reactions because of the occluded skin contact with the chemical.

CLINICAL PRESENTATION

Table 2-4 provides a fairly complete clinical classification[6] of irritation. Previously, ICD was considered a monomorphous process, but it has now been shown to be a complex biologic entity with its own pathophysiology, natural history, and clinical appearance. The actual presentation depends upon multiple internal and external factors.

Acute Irritant Dermatitis

The classic symptoms of skin irritation are often seen when the offending agent is potent and there is sufficient exposure time. This contact with a

TABLE 2-4 Clinical Types of Irritation

Acute irritant dermatitis
Irritant reaction
Delayed acute irritant dermatitis
Cumulative irritant contact dermatitis
Traumatic irritant dermatitis
Pustular and acneiform dermatitis
Nonerythematous irritation
Friction

Source: Data from Ref. 6.

strong primary irritant is often accidental, and the resulting dermatitis is elicited in almost anyone exposed. This cutaneous eruption usually heals soon after exposure, without significant scarring.

Irritant Reaction

The pre-eczematous expression of acute skin irritation is known as an *irritant reaction* and is seen in individuals who are extensively exposed to various irritants. Hairdressers and other wet-work employees frequently develop this type of reaction from frequent exposure.

Delayed, Acute Irritant Dermatitis

Certain chemicals produce acute irritation in a delayed fashion, but the clinical appearance and course of the skin reactions resemble those of acute ICD. Since the onset of symptoms is delayed, patch testing should be performed to separate this entity from ACD.

Cumulative Irritant Contact Dermatitis

When an acute irritant reaction develops from repeated exposure, the resulting dermatitis tends to last longer and to become chronic. The classic signs of this reaction are erythema and dryness followed by hyperkeratosis and fissure formation. This is probably the most common type of ICD that develops after prolonged, subtle exposure to chemical substances. Patch testing is again indicated to avoid confusion with allergic reactions.

Traumatic Irritant Dermatitis

Acute trauma to the skin always precedes traumatic irritant dermatitis. The clinical course may resemble that of a nummular eczema which begins with erythema, vesicles, and scaling followed by a prolonged period of healing. This may occur after a burn or laceration, as well as with an acute irritant dermatitis. The chronicity and recalcitrance of this reaction are similar to those of factitial dermatitis, since the healing phase may be followed by exacerbation.

Pustular and Acneiform Irritant Dermatitis

Exposure to oils, grease, tar, asphalt, or naphthalenes promotes the gradual development of pustular and acneiform irritant dermatitis. This is actually a rare reaction that may depend upon constitutional and individual chemical factors.

Nonerythematous Irritation

In the early phase of skin irritation, subtle skin damage may develop without evidence of visible inflammation. It has been suggested that consumer dissatisfaction with many products may result from exposure to this low-grade irritation. Subjective irritation (stinging, burning, itching, tingling) can occur in some individuals without evidence of irritant contact dermatitis.

Friction Irritation

A moderate degree of friction in everyday life is usually harmless, but chronic friction may induce lichenification of the skin. Friction blisters are well-known responses to sudden mechanical trauma.

The different clinical pictures of acute and chronic irritation can be explained in part by their effects on what has been called the *irritation threshold*.[22,23] With exposure to strong irritants, either the skin is irritated below this threshold and no clinical reaction results or the irritation exceeds the threshold and dermatitis results. When the irritant is weak but the exposure is repetitive, a longer period of time is required to exceed the threshold, but dermatitis eventually develops. The damaged skin now has a lowered threshold which is easier to exceed even with occasional exposure to the irritant.

DIAGNOSTIC CRITERIA

Table 2-5 summarizes a proposed standardization of the difficult diagnosis of ICD.[24] The subjective and objective categories noted have been weighted for major and minor findings, but no arbitrary number of these features need be present to establish the diagnosis. Obviously, the more features one can identify, the stronger the case for ICD. The patch testing procedures utilized to aid in the diagnosis of ACD are discussed in Chapter 4.

Various predisposing factors are important in evaluating the patient sus-

TABLE 2-5 Diagnostic Criteria of ICD

Subjective	
Major	*Minor*
1. Onset of symptoms within minutes to hours of exposure.	1. Onset of dermatitis within 2 weeks of exposure.
2. Pain, burning, stinging, or discomfort exceeding itching early in the clinical course.	2. Many people in the environment affected similarly.

Objective	
Major	*Minor*
1. Macular erythema, hyperkeratosis, or fissuring predominating over vesiculation.	1. Sharp circumspection of the dermatitis.
2. Glazed, parched, or scalded appearance of the epidermis.	2. Evidence of gravitational influence, such as a dripping effect.
3. Healing process begins promptly on withdrawal of exposure to the offending agent.	3. Lack of tendency of the dermatitis to spread.
4. Patch testing is negative.	4. Morphologic changes suggesting small concentration differences or contact time produce large differences in skin damage.

Source: Data from Ref. 16.

pected of having an irritant reaction. Anatomic differences, for instance, make the exposure site very important, since skin permeability is greatest in thin skin areas such as the scrotum or eyelids.[25] The threshold for skin irritation is decreased in children up to age 8 and again in the elderly. Older skin has lower barrier activity with greater stratum corneum permeability.[26]

While it has been a common belief that Caucasians are more susceptible to irritants than African-Americans, this theory is now in question. Studies with transepidermal water loss suggest that black skin may be more susceptible to irritation than white skin.[27–29]

Is a woman's skin more irritation prone than a man's? Irritant dermatitis is certainly more common in women, but prospective studies indicate that any objective differences are small.[30,31] It is more likely that women, because they use a greater number of cosmetic and skin care products and more often perform tasks requiring household cleaning products, are exposed to irritants more frequently than men.

Subjects with pre-existing skin diseases such as atopic dermatitis seem to have an increased susceptibility to irritant reactions. This may be due to a reduced cutaneous threshold to the chemical irritant, inherent xerosis from increased transepidermal water loss, dysfunctional sweating, or a high carriage rate of *Staphylococcus aureus*.[3,17]

TABLE 2-6 High-Risk Occupations for Patients with ICD

Baker
Building worker
Canner
Caterer
Cleaner
Cook
Dental assistant and technicians
Engineer
Hairdresser
Florist, Gardener, Horticulturist
Mechanic
Nurse
Printer
Butcher, Meat packer

Source: Data from Ref. 14.

IRRITANTS IN INDUSTRIAL SETTINGS

Knowledge of irritants in various occupations is key to establishing a diagnosis in patients presenting with dermatitis where the occupational setting is suspect.[14] Some occupations are naturally more prone to occupational dermatitis than others. Table 2-6 lists high-risk occupations for ICD.

Of these, hairdressers are more widely studied than other occupations. The remaining occupations are identified as high risk mainly through individual case reports.

Hair care products (Table 2-3) accounted for 25% of the ICD and ACD due to cosmetics reported by the North American Contact Dermatitis Group in 1985.[12,32] Of these products, shampoos are a frequent cause of ICD in hairdressers, particularly apprentice hairdressers, who perform this function more frequently than their instructors.[33] However, there does not appear to be a significant relationship between dermatitis and the frequency with which hairdressers give shampoos.[34]

PREVENTION

Preventing ICD in the workplace is the aim of all physicians concerned with occupational skin disorders. A multidisciplinary approach is necessary to reduce employee exposure to irritants which can lead to lost work time for both the employer and employee. A team effort involving employers, employees, and government officials is essential to a successful implementation of preventive measures. Sometimes active intervention can prevent occupational skin disorders, such as early identification of a hazardous material, recognition of high-risk workers, and use of hazard control.[35,36]

Potentially hazardous materials can be identified by testing all materials prior to their introduction into the workplace. Material Safety Data Sheets are required by law before the use of new chemicals in a work setting. Preemployment screening for the presence of selected skin diseases is helpful in identifying workers who are more likely to develop irritant reactions in the workplace. Control of ventilation, temperature, and humidity in the work environment can produce a comfortable, safe atmosphere that will not only help prevent ICD but actually increase the resistance of the skin to irritants. Good housekeeping, education of workers, and posting of hazard warnings are useful to keep employees fully productive and on the job. Physical barriers in the workplace can also decrease exposure to mechanical particles. The judicious use of gloves, protective clothing, and barrier creams can also help prevent cutaneous contact with potential irritants.[3,37]

THERAPY AND PROGNOSIS

Removal of the offending agent or removal of the worker from continued exposure to the offending agent may result in the alleviation or elimination of ICD. If this can be accomplished, the prognosis is good. However, this is not always practical.

Failing removal of the offending agent, emollient therapy is one of the few treatments the dermatologist or occupational physician can utilize. Until recently, little information was available on the composition of emollient creams and their commercial counterparts, the moisturizers known as *hand and body lotions*. This information is now available,[38] and dermatologists and occupational physicians can use it to help counsel their patients. Since ACD has a high potential to complicate the clinical picture of ICD, the preservative systems of the moisturizers is an essential part of counseling.[39] Once an effective emollient or moisturizer has been selected, there is a good possibility of limiting the impact of ICD in both the worker's occupation and personal life.

CONCLUSION

Over the past decade, more has been written and presented on ICD than ever before. This expanding field of expertise in contact dermatitis now permits more frequent success in treating ICD in the workplace.

REFERENCES

1. Jackson EM, Goldner R: Preface. In Jackson EM, Goldner R (eds): *Irritant Contact Dermatitis*. New York, Marcel Dekker, 1990, pp vii–viii.

2. Jackson EM: The difference between irritation and sensitization. *J Toxicol & Ocular Toxicol* 4(1):1–2, 1985.
3. Marks JG, DeLeo VA: *Contact and Occupational Dermatology.* St Louis, Mosby, 1992, p 241.
4. Baadsgaard O, Wang T: Immune regulation in allergic and irritant skin reactions, *Int J Dermatol* 30:161–172, 1991.
5. Willis CM, Stephens CJM, Wilkinson JD: Selective expression of immune-associated surface antigens by keratinocytes in irritant contact dermatitis. *J of Invest Dermatol* 96:505–511, 1991.
6. Bason M, Lammintausta K, Maibach HI: Irritant dermatitis. In Marzulli FN, Maibach HI (eds): *Dermatotoxicology,* ed 4. New York, Hemisphere, 1991, p 223.
7. Fleming MG, Bergfeld WF: The etiology of irritant contact dermatitis. In Jackson EM, Goldner R (eds): *Irritant Contact Dermatitis.* New York, Marcel Dekker, 1990, p 41.
8. Rycroft RJG: Low humidity occupational dermatoses. *Dermatol Clin* 2:553–560, 1984.
9. Newhouse ML, Tagg B, Pocock SJ: An epidemiological study of workers producing enzyme washing powders. *Lancet* 1(649):689–693, 1970.
10. Malten KE: Cosmetic, the consumer, the factory worker and the occupational physician. *Contact Dermatitis* 1:16–26, 1975.
11. Jackson EM: Substantiating the safety of fragrances and fragranced products. *Cosmetics & Toiletries* 108:43–44, 46, 1993.
12. Eiermann HJ, Larsen WG, Maibach HI, et al: Prospective study of cosmetic reactions: 1977–1980. *J Am Acad Dermatol* 6:909–917, 1982.
13. Adams RM, Maibach HI: A five year study of cosmetic reactions. *J Am Acad Dermatol* 13:1062–1069, 1985.
14. Bruze M, Emmett EA: Occupational exposure to irritants. In Jackson EM, Goldner R (eds): *Irritant Contact Dermatitis.* New York, Marcel Dekker, 1990, p 81.
15. Rycroft RJG, Smith WDL: Low humidity occupational dermatoses. *Contact Dermatitis* 6:488–492, 1980.
16. Feldmann RJ, Maibach HI: Regional variation in percutaneous penetration. *Int J Dermatol* 48:1813–1819, 1967.
17. Shmunes E: Contact dermatitis in atopic individuals. *Dermatol Clin* 2:561–566, 1984.
18. Fisher AA: *Contact Dermatitis,* ed 3. Philadelphia, Lea & Febiger, 1986, p 131.
19. Adams RM: *Occupational Skin Disease,* ed 2. Philadelphia, WB Saunders, 1990, p 578.
20. Coenraads PJ, Bleumink E, Nater JP: Susceptibility to primary irritants, age dependence and relation to contact allergic reactions. *Contact Dermatitis* 1:377–381, 1975.
21. Rycroft RJG, Wilkinson JD: Irritants and sensitizers. In Champion RH, Burton J, Ebling FJG (eds): *Textbook of Dermatology,* ed 5. Oxford, Blackwell Scientific, 1992, p 717.
22. Dahl MV: Chronic irritant contact dermatitis: Mechanisms, variables and differentiation from other forms of contact dermatitis. *Adv Dermatol* 3:261–275, 1988.
23. Malten KE: Thoughts on irritant contact dermatitis. *Contact Dermatitis* 7:238–247, 1981.

REFERENCES

24. Rietschel RL: Diagnosing irritant contact dermatitis. In Jackson EM, Goldner R (eds): *Irritant Contact Dermatitis*. New York, Marcel Dekker, 1990, p 167.
25. Schmunes E: Predisposing factors in occupational skin diseases. *Dermatol Clin* 6:7–13, 1988.
26. Cua AB, Wilhelm KP, Maibach HI: Cutaneous sodium lauryl sulfate irritation potential: Age and regional variability. *Br J Dermatol* 123:607–613, 1990.
27. Kligman AM, Wooding WM: A method for the measurement and evaluation of irritants on human skin. *J Invest Dermatol* 49:78–94, 1967.
28. Weigand DA, Gaylor JR: Irritant reaction in Negro and Caucasian skin. *South Med J* 67:548–551, 1974.
29. Berardesca E, Maibach HI: Racial differences in sodium lauryl sulfate-induced cutaneous irritation: Black and white. *Contact Dermatitis* 18:65–70, 1988.
30. Bjornberg A: Skin reactions to primary irritants in men and women. *Acta Derm Venereol* 55:191–194, 1975.
31. Lammintausta K, Maibach HI, Wilson D: Irritant reactivity in males and females. *Contact Dermatitis* 17:276–280, 1987.
32. Marks JG: Cosmetics. In Adams RM (ed): *Occupational Skin Disease*, ed 2. Philadelphia, WB Saunders, 1993, p 326–348.
33. Cronin E, Kullavanijaya P: Hand dermatitis in hairdressers. *Acta Derm Venereol* 85(Suppl):47–50, 1979.
34. Stovall GK, Levin L, Oler J: Occupational dermatitis among hairdressers. *J Occup Med* 25:871–878, 1983.
35. Mathias CGT: Prevention of occupational contact dermatitis. *J Am Acad Dermatol* 23:742–748, 1990.
36. Tucker SB: Prevention of occupational skin disease. *Dermatol Clin* 6:87–96, 1988.
37. Fisher T: Prevention of irritant dermatitis. In Adams RM (ed): *Occupational Medicine: State of the Art Reviews*. Philadelphia, Hanley and Belfus, 1986, p 335.
38. Jackson EM: Moisturizers: What's in them? How do they work? *Am J Contact Dermatitis* 3:162–168, 1992.
39. Jackson EM: Quaternium-15: Benefit or risk in cosmetics? *Cosmetic Dermatol* 6:37–38, 1993.

3

The Differential Diagnosis of Occupational Dermatoses

Anthony F. Fransway

INTRODUCTION

The skin, like many organ systems, has a limited number of response patterns resulting from a wide variety of exogenous and endogenous stimuli; these include erythema, scaling, hyperkeratosis, fissuring, papulation, vesiculation, edema, and pigmentary change, alone and in various combinations. Yet within these limited response patterns, the intricacy of dermatologic presentations is manifested in myriad combinations of morphology, distribution, and evolution. It is necessary for the proficient occupational dermatologist to recognize the varied presentations of the occupational dermatoses, nonoccupational dermatologic diseases, and various combinations thereof. This chapter summarizes the most frequent pitfalls in differential diagnosis, although a complete synopsis of all skin disorders that might be confused with occupational disease is well beyond its scope and would resemble a standard dermatologic text (Figures 3-1, 3-2, 3-3, and 3-4).

The importance of diagnosing nonoccupational dermatologic problems seems self-evident, but for physicians concentrating on occupational difficulties, it is natural to focus initially on work origins. The vital need to diagnose nonoccupational disease correctly is evident when one considers that occupational dermatoses themselves (even when well defined) frequently respond poorly to avoidance of causative allergens and medical therapy; definition of the nonoccupational component of disease may direct the physician to an alternative treatment program and, with skill and good fortune, to a prefera-

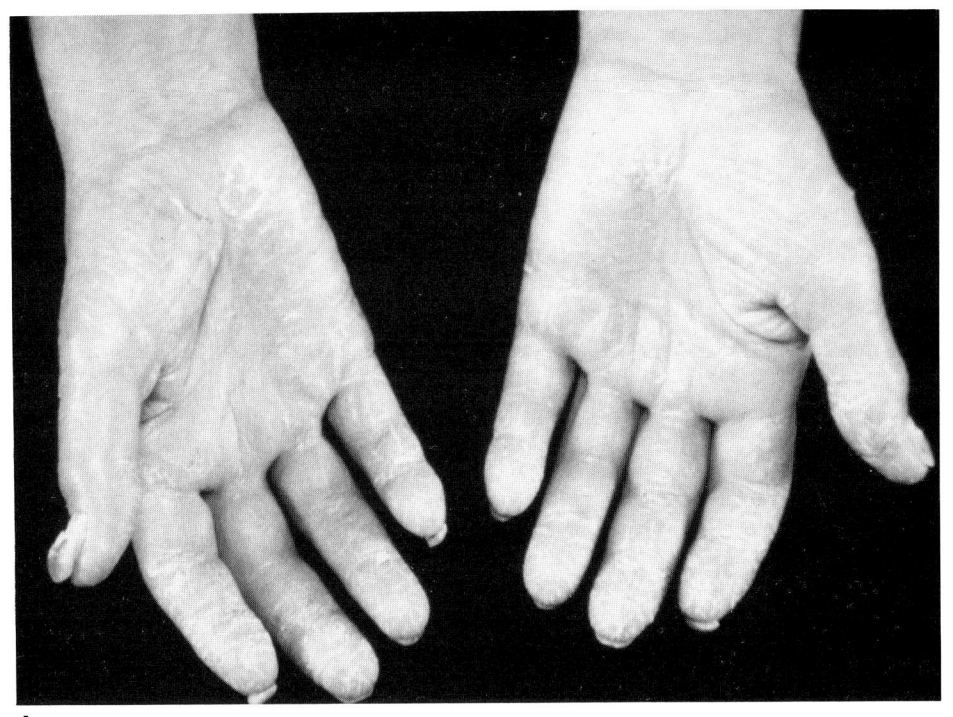

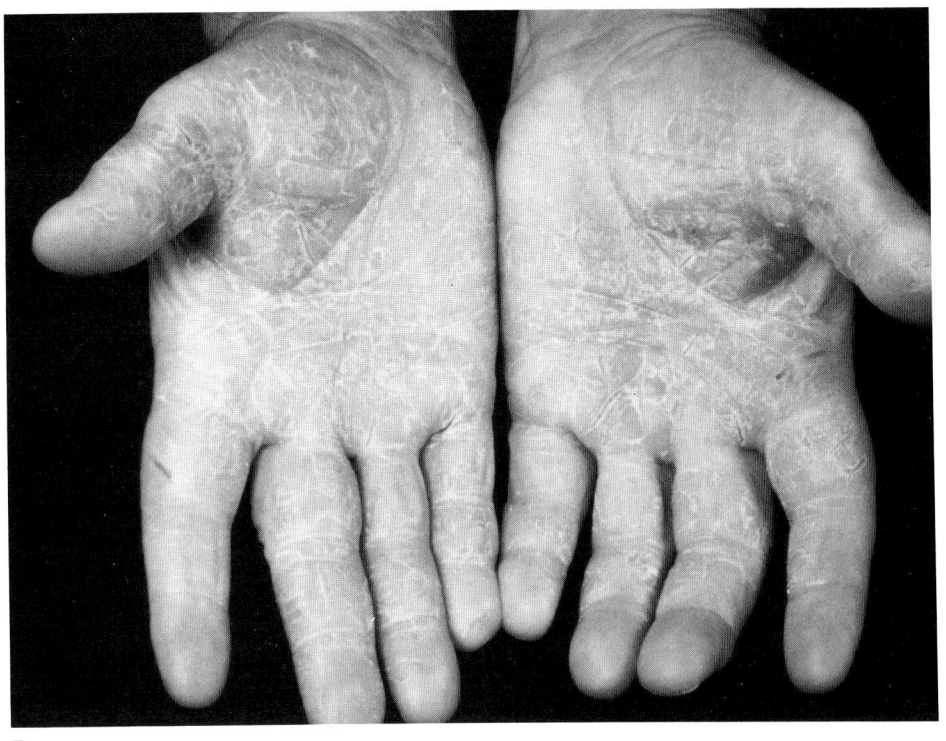

Figure 3-1. a. Psoriasiform keratoderma in a known psoriatic. b. Psoriasiform keratoderma with active dermatitis indistinguishable from that in (a), other than nail involvement, due to occupational chromate exposure and sensitivity.

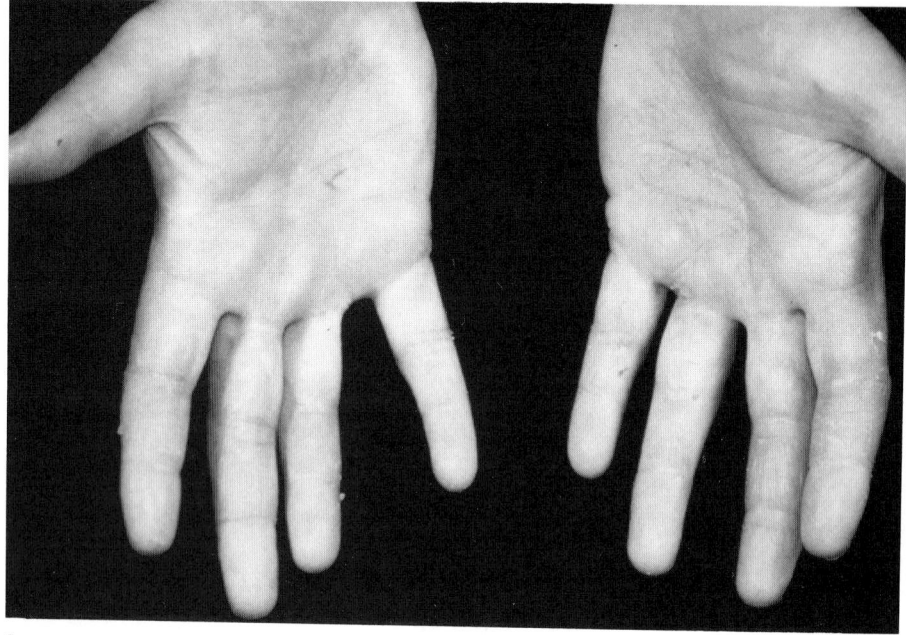

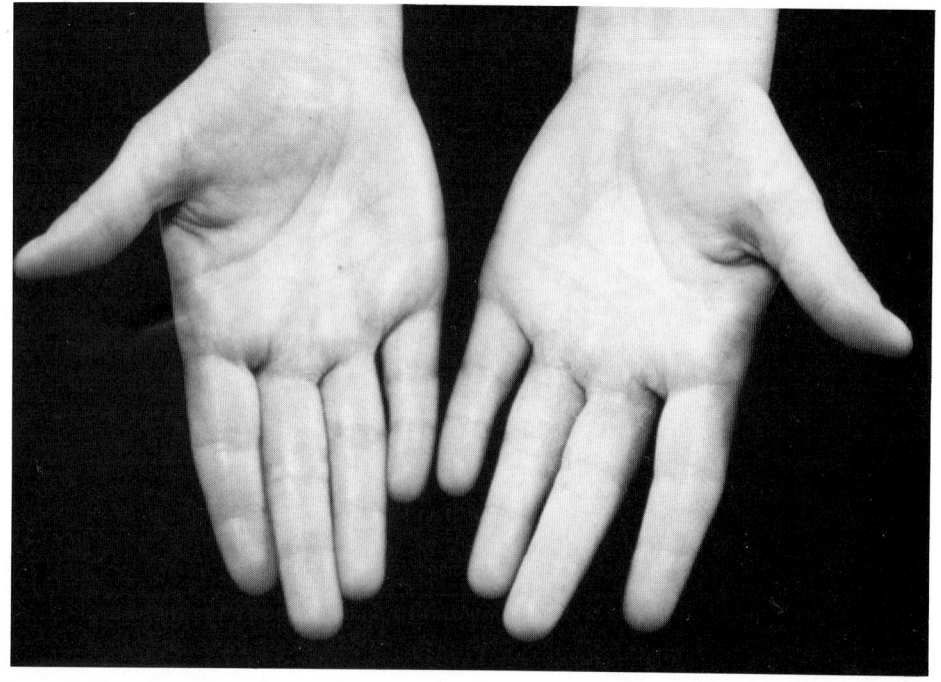

Figure 3-2. a. Patchy dermatitis of the digits and midpalm of atopic origin. b. Patchy dermatitis of the digits and midpalm, with additional dorsal hand involvement; medical technician with allergic contact dermatitis to accelerants used in glove manufacture.

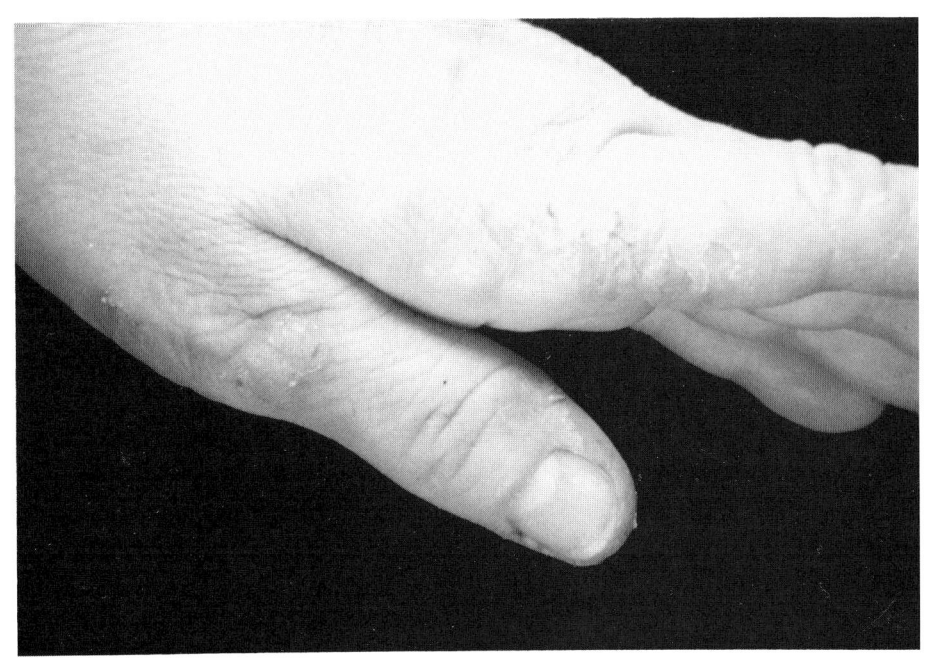

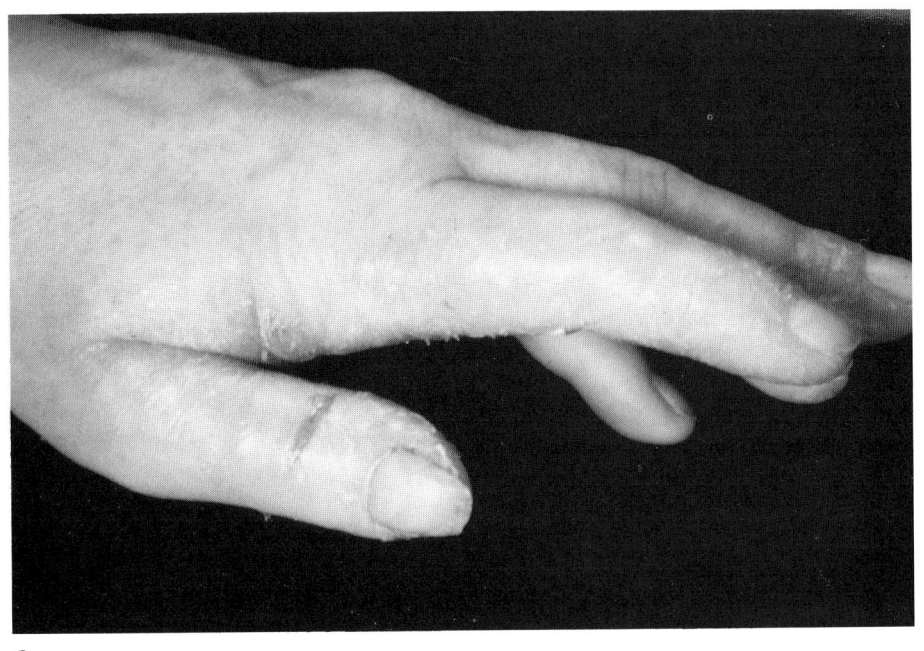

Figure 3-3. a. Impetiginized focal digital eczema of irritant origin. b. Impetiginized focal digital eczema, indistinguishable from that in (a), in a patient with sensitivity and exposure to epoxy resin.

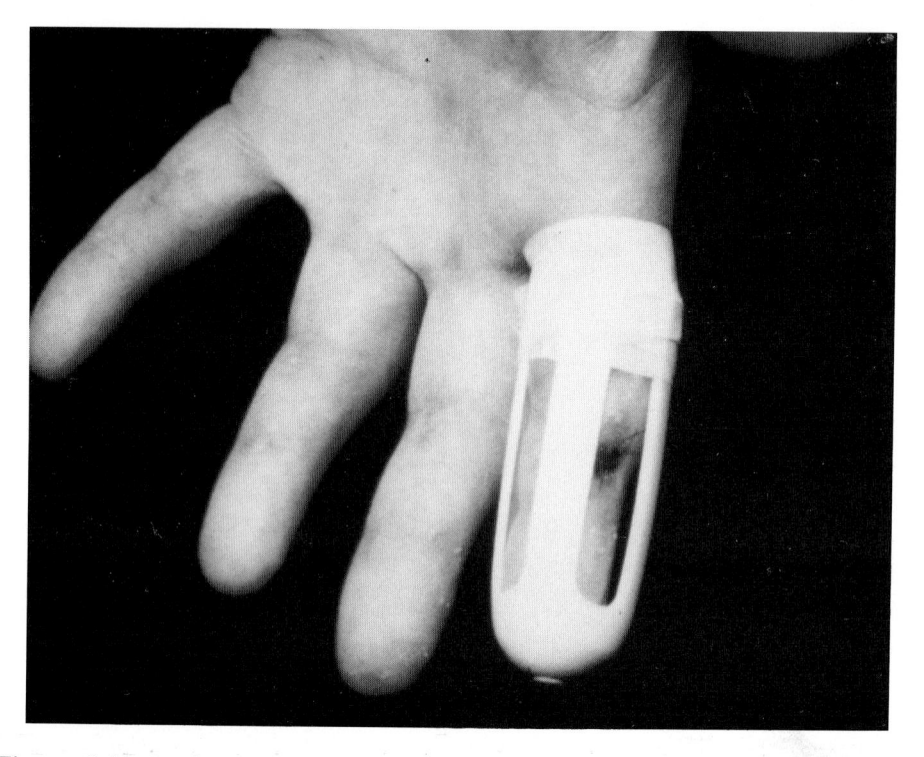

Figure 3-4. Dual-origin digital difficulties. Finger laceration with cast of occupational origin; focal digital and palmar keratoderma of paraneoplastic origin unrelated to the workplace.

ble outcome. Primary dermatologic disease of a nonoccupational nature frequently has more specific and effective therapy and therefore requires recognition for the physician to intervene definitively at the earliest possible juncture.

The consequences of misdiagnosing an occupational dermatosis in the evaluation of such patients include not only failure of evaluation and therapeutic attempts, but social and economic costs as well. The unnecessary and avoidable nature of some workers' compensation, with its attendant expense, litigation, and spent professional energies (not to mention loss of employee productivity), becomes obvious when dealing with the multiply evaluated, extensively tested worker lacking a definitive diagnosis; more far-reaching effects include the psychological impact on other workers performing the same job, who may develop the belief that a workplace problem exists, necessitating visits from a variety of government agencies. Such a scenario highlights the need to correctly and definitively diagnose as early as possible (if not at first contact).

Our task as occupational dermatologists would be greatly simplified if such clear distinction existed in the real world. In fact, the usual case study involves the interaction of numerous factors that play a role in the patient's final dermatologic disease. For example, the development of an occupational dermatosis may be initiated, potentiated, or complicated by the presence of nonoccupational factors, such as a family or personal history of atopic diathesis, psoriasis, and poor hygiene; as evaluating physicians, we are additionally called upon to determine which dermatosis came first and what is the primary component of the patient's difficulty. Second, the relative contributions of occupational and nonoccupational factors often comes into question even when allergic contact dermatitis is clearly defined. One can envision many illustrative examples, such as the carpenter who "does it himself" at home or the sensitized machinist who also has pertinent ongoing home exposures (e.g., formaldehyde-donating biocides and isothiazolinone derivatives in household and personal-care products). Identifying the initial inciting event is crucial in determining whether an occupational dermatosis *sui generis* exists or whether the patient with nonoccupational sensitivity is also exposed to the same antigen family in the work environment.

Yet other variables complicate the issue. The problem occasionally becomes one of definition of terms, as we have all painfully learned when asked to testify on the relative role of job stress in the worsening of endogenous or exogenous disease or to determine whether posttraumatic eczema represents a true occupational phenomenon or merely an epiphenomenon.[1] In the real world, although clear-cut, straightforward cases of occupational allergic contact or irritant contact dermatitis do occur, often it is a continuum of participating environmental, occupational, and nonoccupational exposures to which the occupational dermatologist must assign relative importance.

The exclusion of an occupational origin for a given dermatosis and the diagnosis of alternative primary dermatologic disease is by definition dependent on the exclusion of an occupational source, and may rely on the use of a number of techniques and investigational procedures; these must include a detailed history and physical examination, and may include biopsy for histology, direct immunofluorescence or electron microscopy, microbiologic culture, and certainly inclusive epicutaneous patch testing in the majority of patients. It is only through the definition of all contributing variables that the optimal outcome for the patient may be achieved.

The majority of occupational dermatoses involve hand eczema and other extremity conditions; this review will, of necessity, concentrate on those acral dermatoses that may be confused with work-related disease; other dermatologic presentations and distributions will be reviewed as relevant and feasible. As a physical examination is often paramount in developing an initial index of suspicion, a morphologic classification of differential diagnosis has been adopted by the author (Table 3-1).

NONOCCUPATIONAL DERMATOSES

Papulosquamous Dermatoses

Psoriasis

One of the most frequent pitfalls in the distinction of nonoccupational dermatoses is that of diagnosing palmar/palmoplantar psoriasis. Psoriasis of the

TABLE 3-1 Differential Diagnosis of Occupational Dermatoses

- I. Papulosquamous dermatoses
    - A. Psoriasis and variant pustular dermatoses
    - B. Lichen planus
    - C. Tinea manuum
    - D. Dermal reticulosis/cutaneous T-cell lymphoma
    - E. Ichthyoses
- II. Eczema/dermatitis
    - A. Exogenous
        1. Irritant
        2. Allergic
        3. Contact urticaria
        4. Actinic dermatitis
    - B. Endogenous
        1. Atopic eczema
        2. Dyshidrosis/pompholyx
        3. Nummular eczema
        4. Seborrheic dermatitis
        5. Rosacea-like dermatitis
- III. Keratodermas
    - A. Hereditary
    - B. Frictional/reactive/irritant
    - C. Endogenous/hormonal/paraneoplastic
- IV. Infectious/acneiform
    - A. Fungal
    - B. Bacterial
    - C. Viral
    - D. Atypical mycobacterial
- V. Vesicobullous
    - A. Epidermolysis bullosa, hereditary and acquired
    - B. Pemphigus/pemphigoid
    - C. Porphyria cutanea tarda
- VI. Pigmentary
    - A. Vitiligo
    - B. Postinflammatory hyperpigmentation and hypopigmentation
- VII. Atypical/bizarre
    - A. Factitial
    - B. Malingering
    - C. Manipulative
    - D. Psychiatric disease/delusions of parasitosis
    - E. Neuropathic
- VIII. Miscellaneous
    - A. Alcohol and drug abuse

hands frequently presents as sharply marginated, slightly erythematous patches with firmly adherent yellow scales and callus formation preferentially involving the palms, with relative dorsal sparing; the fissuring and hyperkeratosis present in such plaques often makes the distinction from hyperkeratotic eczema impossible.[2] The decision on whether a significant occupational precipitating factor exists is dependent upon an exhaustive history, as psoriatic patients without frictional trauma are much less likely to have occupationally exacerbated disease than are those with a demonstrable Koebner phenomenon; Fisher's case of frictional trauma in a pharmacist caused by unscrewing prescription container caps is an excellent example of an occult occupational factor worsening nonoccupational disease.[3] Similarly, the overweight salesperson with plantar psoriasis from prolonged standing and walking is another subtle example. More often, the distinction requires extensive epicutaneous patch testing, as in the case of the cement worker with significant frictional/irritant factors who also has chromium sensitivity as a primary component of hyperkeratotic psoriasiform palmar disease. Many other examples may be cited, such as the typist with psoriasis and Koebnerized nail dystrophy and the development of periungual erythema in psoriatics employed in wet-work occupations.[4,5]

Although the percentage of psoriatics with localized palmar and plantar disease is quite small, psoriasis is a highly prevalent condition (with 3 to 7 million individuals so affected in the United States alone); this in part explains the frequent need to distinguish psoriasis and psoriasiform occupational dermatitis. The sharp demarcation of psoriatic plaques on the palms may be helpful, as may the relative absence of pruritus.

Conditions accepted as probably variant psoriatic presentations, such as palmoplantar pustulosis or papulovesicular dermatosis of the palms and soles, may also be difficult to differentiate from vesicular occupational irritant or allergic dermatitis. A history of chronicity and the distribution of disease (the central palm and the instep of the sole) may be helpful in making the distinction; when widespread vesicles and pruritus predominate, inclusive patch tests and skin biopsy generally serve to clarify the situation.

The relative role of ingestion of nickel or chromium in occupationally sensitized individuals in the flaring of pustular and vesicular hand dermatoses is arguable and requires clarification; at least some investigators feel that ingestion of such antigens is important in dermatosis propagation.[6,7] As nickel and chromium are ubiquitous antigens both at home and in the workplace, the relative contribution of occupational, casual, and dietary exposures may demand attention.

As in other hand dermatoses, the final distinction of endogenous palmar psoriasis versus occupational contact dermatitis often relies upon the results of epicutaneous patch testing. In the experience of this author, biopsy of the palm to distinguish psoriasis is invariably fruitless, with eczema and psoriasis alike showing simple changes of psoriasiform hyperplasia and dermatitic spongiosis; such biopsy is not advocated without a more widespread distribution of disease, in which case it may not be needed. If a skin biopsy is indicated, biopsy of a nonpalmar lesion is more likely to be diagnostic.

Lichen Planus

Lichen planus is a disease quite similar to psoriasis with respect to the approach of the occupational dermatologist, as its propensity to exhibit an isomorphic phenomenon and its definition as a psychocutaneous syndrome with a stress flare factor raise potential occupational issues even without contact sensitization. Occupational lichenoid reactions such as those seen with sensitivity to photographic chemicals and to gold make the exclusion of allergy to potential contact antigens occasionally necessary.[8,9] As 10 of Altman and Perry's 307 patients with lichen planus at the Mayo Clinic exhibited palmar and/or palmar and plantar disease, a complete physical examination, skin biopsy (very helpful in this setting), and exclusion of relevant contact allergens by patch testing are important and definitive techniques in diagnosis clarification.[10]

Tinea Manuum

Sharply demarcated, scaly hyperkeratosis with minimal pruritus and limited erythema are characteristics of palmar dermatophytosis, a condition which may be occupationally predisposed by humid or moist working conditions, occlusion, and excessive perspiration. Unilateral or asymmetrical involvement aids in making the diagnosis (the so-called two-foot, one-hand syndrome), which is confirmed through microscopic examination of a potassium hydroxide preparation and a mycologic culture.

Dermal Reticulosis

Fixed, sharply demarcated, indurated or infiltrated, painful, or pruritic plaques of the palms and soles, unresponsive to standard modalities of therapy, may suggest the diagnosis of a precursor to T-cell lymphoma occasionally referred to as *dermal reticulosis*. This disease is morphologically psoriasiform. The only clinical clue to the diagnosis may be the induration at the periphery of active lesions. Histologic examination is confirmatory, although a dermatopathologist experienced in detection of subtle cytologic and architectural changes is a requirement. As this is a relatively rare dermatologic condition, the exclusion of more common dermatoses, including contact dermatitis and psoriasis, is required, as may be a longitudinal study to document progressive, more generalized disease with time.

More controversial is the issue of whether occupational dermatoses, chronic dermatitis, or chronic contact sensitivity may be precursor states for cutaneous T-cell lymphoma and of whether transitional states exist. The issue of chronic antigenic stimulation and/or persistence as contributory to the development of mycosis fungoides has been reviewed; clinical evidence has focused on the finding of multiple contact sensitivities in patients with cutaneous T-cell lymphoma, and histologically, the characterization of lymphomatoid contact dermatitis (a benign condition with the histologic features of lymphomatoid malignancy) is interesting.[11-15] Although rare cases of histologically verified benign dermatitis with subsequent development of mycosis fungoides have been documented in the literature, further study is required before any link between chronic antigenic stimulation and cutaneous T-cell malignancies can be suggested.[16,17] The finding of lymphoid tumorigenesis in a small percentage of rodents sensitized and chronically exposed to metal allergens is provocative but not verified.[18]

Ichthyoses

The hyperkeratosis and scaly exfoliation of ichthyosis vulgaris are rarely a problem in distinguishing this disease from occupational dermatosis, although workplace conditions including the low-humidity occupational environment may worsen preexistent disease. Ichthyotic dermatoses severe enough to affect the arms, hands, neck and face (airborne distribution) are easily discerned from the history, clinical findings on physical examination, and histologic examination if necessary.

Eczema/Dermatitis

In no clinical circumstance or expression of disease is a multifactorial etiology as important as it is in hand dermatitis. Because of the multiple compounding factors, the argument of occupational as opposed to nonoccupational dermatosis often hinges upon the "most proximal cause" of difficulty, but the resolution or improvement of the problem is dependent on attention to *all* involved factors. This was recognized some time ago by Lane and colleagues, who felt that contact dermatitis, physical and thermal trauma, secondary bacterial and fungal infection, exposure to soap and irritants, trauma, vascular and hormonal factors, seasonal variation, and distant infectious nidus are important factors in the development of the final common pathway, infectious eczematoid dermatitis.[19] To a degree, it becomes an issue of classification, with Rycroft identifying atopic, seborrheic, and nummular eczema as strictly nonoccupational, even in occupational settings with constant frictional and potentially precipatory trauma.[20] DeBoer and colleagues see the issue differently, classifying the dyshidrotic eczema seen in a significant number of metal workers without contact hypersensitivity as occupational.[21] As the prevalence of hand dermatitis to some degree (classified as endogenous versus exogenous) has been found to vary between 1.2% and 44% by different authors and in different studies, it is important to account for nonoccupational factors in all circumstances of hand eczema.[22-24]

Exogenous Eczema/Dermatoses

Irritant Dermatitis. Although some authors suggest further subclassification, cases of irritant contact dermatitis may be separated into those with an acute or chronic insult origin, with the acute form rarely a problem diagnostically due to the causative, often single overwhelming external exposure. Chronic irritant dermatitis, on the other hand, may involve a variety of both obvious and subtle factors, including irritant chemicals in and out of the workplace, dry environmental conditions and low-humidity occupational and nonoccupational dermatoses, proximity to moving air, and friction. Seasonal variation, with exposure to excessively cold and dry air, may induce xerosis, chapping, and erythema of the hands and face that may be mistaken for occupational disease; similarly, conditions of high humidity may predispose to acneiform eruptions, folliculitis, and fissuring and peeling due to perspiration, evaporation, and subsequent dehydration (as in juvenile plantar dermatosis). Although all of these factors may be occupational, similar nonworkplace exposures abound and must be figured into any equation. The identification of all potential irritants and the protection of exposed skin are mandatory for improvement of dermatosis, as well as in avoiding confusion of primary occupational disease with attendant workers' compensation pursuit.[25-27]

Allergic Contact Dermatitis of Nonoccupational Origin. Familiarity with the need to exclude this entity makes only brief mention necessary. Certain antigens, by the nature of their exposural characteristics, are strictly or primarily occupational, making distinction a simple matter of history taking, testing, and correlation. For other antigens, the relative roles of workplace and leisure-time exposures may be in question and may even be impossible to delineate with adequate certainty; formaldehyde and its derivatives, fragrances, and nickel are obvious examples. Ubiquitous substances such as these require apportionment of work and nonwork exposures in dermatitis propagation, a difficult task made harder when one considers exotic antigen sources such as dietary nickel and balsam of Peru (as previously mentioned, implicated by some in the propagation of hand dermatitis). Practically, this distinction may be a moot point, as complete avoidance of the antigen is often required for dermatitis improvement.[28]

Contact Urticaria. Again requiring only passing mention, contact urticaria is generally easily excluded or included through a history and exposural review, as in latex hypersensitivity in health care workers and contact urticaria to acidic foods and spices in caterers. Several ingredients of moisturizers or cosmetic products, such as sorbic acid, may induce stinging or contact urticaria and thus need to be distinguished from contact urticants of occupational origin.

Dermatoheliosis. Actinically damaged skin, slowly acquired either on the job or at leisure (or both), may occasionally be mistaken for occupational dermatitis if pruritus is a prominent feature, if manipulation causes pruriginized nodules or secondary lichen simplex chronicus, or if the evaluating physician is unfamiliar with the many changes seen with chronic sun exposure. A 41-year-old mechanic I recently evaluated serves as an example. His was a workman's compensation case evaluated by several physicians, in which the only clinical findings were those of actinically damaged skin, pruriginized nodules, and hyperkeratosis; no primary dermatologic disease or occupational sensitizer was identified, biopsy confirmed the clinical suspicion, and the case was rapidly settled.

Endogenous Eczema

Atopic/Dyshidrotic Eczema

Minor forms of atopic eczema, particularly those localized to the hands and fingers in adults, may not only be confused with occupational dermatitis (irritant or allergic) but may also be compounded and worsened by occupational exposures, including irritants and chemicals, occlusion, and perspiration. Scaly erythema with inflammation, fissuring, and subsequent hypopigmentation asymmetrically, in focal fashion, suggests this diagnosis. When impetiginized and sharply localized, atopic eczema may present as nummular eczema, yet another dermatosis that may be confused with occupational disease. As allergic contact dermatitis may also manifest in nummular fashion, patch testing to exclude relevant antigens is necessary before arriving at the diagnoses of atopic or nummular hand eczema of a nonoccupational nature.[29,30]

Dyshidrotic eczema, or pompholyx, is an acute or chronic vesicular response of the hands and feet, frequently localized to the lateral aspects of the palms and fingers; a prodrome of pruritus and burning is common. As the onset may be acute and eruptive, the issue of precipitating factors and/or contact allergen exposure frequently arises, in spite of its rather typical clinical appearance. Psychological stresses, bacterial infection, ingested medications, ingested metals, xerosis, and sweat gland dysfunction have all been implicated in the etiopathogenesis of pompholyx, as has allergic contact dermatitis.[31] Although Meneghini and Angelini found that 30% of their dyshidrotic eczema patients had positive patch test reactions, other investigators have found this to be much less frequent in comparison to patch testing in other eczematous states. Contact allergen assessment may again be required to fully exclude contact sensitization, and irritant factors need to be addressed to minimize their role in dyshidrosis propagation and precipitation.[21,32,33]

Asteatotic/Xerotic Eczema

Rarely is this entity a problem in the differential diagnosis of occupational dermatitis. A purely asteatotic (nonirritant) condition adequate to cause clinical xerosis of the hands is most frequently associated with the findings of erytheme cracquelé of the extremities and noninflammatory scaly desquamation. Irritant factors need to be excluded.

Seborrheic Dermatitis

Allergic contact dermatitis of occupational or nonoccupational origin may mimic seborrheic dermatitis on occasion, especially if modified by the use of topical corticosteroids, with resultant masking of erythema and edema. Although the distribution of seborrheic dermatitis is rather typical, erythema of the periocular and perioral regions may appear seborrheiform while actually stemming from contact sensitivity. Patch testing, sometimes required, excludes this possibility.[34]

More difficult to assess is the fleeting erythematous, slightly exfoliative zygomatic dermatitis that has been proposed to be associated with exposure to video display terminals, intermittently characterized morphologically as rosacea-like or in a seborrheic distribution. Indeed, Liden has demonstrated eloquently that the vast majority of such "VDT dermatitis" cases actually represent a diverse group of nonoccupational disorders including seborrheic dermatitis, rosacea, and allergic and irritant contact dermatitis.[35] In studying over 300 office workers at the Mayo Clinic exposed to computer video terminals for a mean period of over 20 hours per week, no cases of "terminal" dermatitis were identified; acne, quiescent rosacea, and other unrelated dermatologic and nondermatologic disorders were identified based on the history and physical examination of this cohort.[36] The role of static electricity in the impaction of particulate matter on the faces of such workers has been questioned, without confirmation to date. Yet the issue has again been recently resurrected, and further study may be needed to put this issue and this entity to rest.[37]

Keratodermas

This diverse group of dermatoses, with the final common pathways of palmar and plantar hyperkeratosis and acanthosis, may be associated with hereditary, endogenous and paraneoplastic, and frictional or reactive components. Morphologic examination and a history of disease onset help define endogenous factors such as paraneoplasia and endocrinologic disorders as contributory, while family and personal histories are generally adequate for the distinction of hereditary keratodermas. Frictional or reactive keratodermas are frequently occupationally based, although rarely a cause of significant disability and often not reported by the worker. Irritant factors in the workplace may unmask a hereditary subclinical keratoderma, but again, significant morbidity is unusual.

Infectious/Acneiform Dermatoses

A variety of infectious disorders may cause occasional confusion with respect to occupational dermatitis, but generally these conditions as a group are relatively easily excluded by their clinical appearance, a potassium hydroxide preparation, and appropriate cultures; in rare cases, histologic examination may be helpful. More difficult is the problem of secondary bacterial, viral, or fungal invasion of a preexistent occupational or nonoccupational hand dermatosis, where a high index of suspicion is paramount in making the correct diagnosis.

Tinea pedis et manuum, as discussed previously, rarely causes a diagnostic dilemma. Occasionally more difficult to distinguish is the dermatophytid reaction to a chronic cutaneous focus of tinea, which often appears dyshidrotic, acute, and vesicular and may be confused with acute contact dermatitis.[38] The presence of secondary invasion by *Candida albicans* may also be difficult to discern in the background of chronic dermatitis (endogenous or exogenous origin). Cultures again are confirmatory.

The pathogenetic role of bacteria in the flaring of a dermatitic focus, particularly hand eczema, seems to be undisputed despite the lack of definitive evidence. Supportive is the presence of various gram-negative and particularly gram-positive species when culture is performed, the rapid improvement of impetiginized hand eczema when treated with systemic antibiotics, and the implicated immunopathogenesis of the bacterid and dermatophytid. Primary impetigo of the hands may mimic nummular or allergic contact eczema but may be distinguished by the morphology of the erythematous patches with honey-colored crusts or bullous change, again confirmed by culture.

Acneiform eruptions (see Chapter 8), when exhibiting the typical appearance of comedones and papules, rarely cause difficulty in the distinction from occupational disease. The role of a work environment in which perspiration, exogenous oils and greases, and humidity are excessive is uncertain, but at least a subgroup of acne vulgaris patients do suffer from such exogenous vectors, worsening the endogenous tendency. When acne with predominant pustules is seen, particularly when extensive and monomorphous in the background of preceding chronic oral antibiotic therapy, the possibility of gram-negative acne exists; such a morphologic presentation may be confused with the occupational dermatosis chloracne, caused by exposure to hydrocarbons such as dioxin. Performance of culture, a history of antibiotic administration, and a history of chemical exposure in the workplace generally distinguish the two conditions adequately.

Herpetic infection may represent an occupational dermatosis, as in herpes gladiatorum in wrestlers or herpetic whitlow in the lacerated or abraded fingers of health care workers (see Chapter 8). Secondary infection of preexistent eczema, either endogenous or exogenous in origin, may mimic an acute contact dermatitis flare; a high index of suspicion is required to diagnose so-called eczema herpeticum. Vacciniform or umbilicated vesicular morphology and the pain that occasionally accompanies such lesions are of assistance. Viral culture, shell vial assay, or immunofluorescent assay are confirmatory. Milker's nodule and orf are additional viral occupational dermatoses to consider.

Vesicobullous Disease

Immunobullous dermatoses of the palms and soles, particularly when localized exclusively to these locations, may occasionally be difficult to distinguish from acute contact dermatitis and dyshidrosis. More frequently, the generalized involvement in disorders such as bullous pemphigoid, pemphigus or epidermolysis bullosa acquisita, and the milia, hypertrichosis, and pigmentary change of porphyria cutanea tarda make such distinction simpler. The congenital bullous dermatoses such as epidermolysis bullosa typically involve either a family history of similar disease or a disease preceding occupational placement that makes their diagnosis possible, although latent cases may be worsened or precipitated by workplace trauma (particularly if one marches for a living!). Biopsy with direct immunofluorescence and histologic study, indirect immunofluorescence, and, rarely, electron microscopy may be helpful in certain circumstances.

Pigmentary Disorders

Although many pigmentary disorders may occasionally be questioned as occupational in nature, the most common disease in which a workplace component or role is confirmed is occupational vitiligo. The complicating issue involves the finding of depigmentation in sites distant from the chemical exposure, with generalized and bilateral disease much like autoimmune, generalized, symmetrical vitiligo. In such circumstances, a family history and a past medical history of such disease, as well as the temporal association of depigmentation with exposure to a chemical capable of such pigment destruction, is required.[39] Benzene derivatives such as catechols and phenols are the most frequently implicated agents, particularly if group substitution occurs in the para position. The problem of determining the relevance of chemical exposure in a patient with preexistent vitiligo occasionally arises, highlighting the need for a complete preemployment physical prior to entry into an at-risk occupation. There is no question that individual susceptibility to chemical depigmentation exists, as has been demonstrated by several investigators (see Chapter 8).[40]

Postinflammatory hyperpigmentation and hypopigmentation may result from any inflammatory dermatologic disease or process, is more common in more deeply pigmented individuals, and requires characterization and definition of the underlying dermatosis to assess the occupational significance. Melasma in the outdoor worker exposed to chemicals that are airborne or sprayed may rarely cause confusion.

Atypical/Bizarre Diseases

The atypical or bizarre skin condition claimed to be of occupational origin may be suspected on the basis of several morphologic features. These include nonhealing ulcerative or erosive disease; ulceration with angulated, linear, or punched-out edges; excoriation; and peculiar disease not typical of any known dermatosis. Such factitial disease may be a conscious attempt to deceive the physician to obtain occupational compensation and disability pay (as in the case of malingering) or may be a manifestation of a more serious, deeply rooted psychopathology (such as Secretan's syndrome and Munchausen's syndrome).[41]

Other psychiatric dermatoses, such as monosymptomatic delusional hypochondriasis (delusions of parasitosis), generally declare themselves through the patient's fixed and rigid belief in a specific origin despite evidence to the contrary. I have seen cases of fixed delusional belief regarding parasitic infestation in employees exposed to coworkers with scabies or other ectoparasites severe enough to require psychiatric consultation in one circumstance. Such assistance may be invaluable in cases without a clear-cut alternative explanation.

Other atypical presentations may represent manifestations of alcohol or drug abuse, which need to be considered in certain circumstances.

SUMMARY AND CONCLUSIONS

The above is a brief overview of several dermatoses that may mimic occupational dermatoses and is not intended to represent a complete summary or exhaustive review of all potential scenarios. In addition to increasing the dermatologist's index of suspicion, it is the hope of the author that this review has highlighted the importance of considering multiple factors in a given dermatologic disease presentation, as well as the need to consider the presenting dermatosis as the endpoint of numerous interacting factors with varying occupational and nonoccupational relevance. Clear-cut distinction in a situation of purely occupational or purely endogenous origin approaches perfection, which is rarely part of the human experience. The exclusion and inclusion of all factors in a given dermatosis are required to be most effective as an occupational dermatologist.

REFERENCES

1. Mathias CGT: Post-traumatic eczema. *Dermatol Clin* 6:35–42, 1988.
2. Braun Falco O, Plegwig G, Wolff HH, et al: Erythematous and erythreosquamous skin diseases. In *Dermatology*. Heidelberg, Springer-Verlag, 1991, p 425.
3. Fisher AA: Occupational palmar psoriasis due to safety prescription container caps. *Contact Dermatitis* 1:56, 1979.
4. Schmunes E: Predisposing factors in occupational skin diseases. *Dermatol Clin* 6:7–13, 1988.
5. Scher RK: Occupational nail disorders. *Dermatol Clin* 6:27–34, 1988.
6. Veien NK: Systemically induced eczema in adults. *Acta Derm Venereol* (Suppl 147):1–58, 1989.
7. Christensen OB, Lindstrom C, Lufberg H, et al: Micromorphology and specificity of oral induced flare-ups in nickel sensitive patients. *Acta Derm Venereol* 61:505–510, 1981.
8. Knudsen E: Lichen planus-like eruption caused by color developer. *Arch Dermatol* 89:357–360, 1964.
9. Buckley WR: Lichenoid eruptions following contact dermatitis. *Arch Dermatol* 78:454–458, 1958.
10. Altman J, Perry HO: The variations and course of lichen planus. *Arch Dermatol* 84:47–59, 1961.
11. Tan RSH, Butterworth CM, McLaughlin H, et al: Mycosis fungoides—a disease of antigen persistence. *Br J Dermatol* 91:607–616, 1974.
12. Lambert WC: Premycotic eruptions. *Dermatol Clin* 3:629–645, 1985.
13. Shupp DL, Winkelmann RK: Patch tests in Sezary syndrome and mycosis fungoides. *Contact Dermatitis* 13:180–185, 1985.
14. Orbaneja JG, Diaz LI, Lozano JLS, et al: Lymphomatoid contact dermatitis. *Contact Dermatitis* 2:139–143, 1976.
15. Ecker RI, Winkelmann RK: Lymphomatoid contact dermatitis. *Contact Dermatitis* 7:84–93, 1981.

16. Fransway AF, Winkelmann RK: Chronic dermatitis evolving to mycosis fungoides: report of four cases and review of the literature. *Cutis* 41:330–335, 1988.
17. Whittemore AS, Holly EA, I-M Lee: Mycosis fungoides in relation to environmental exposure and immune response: A case-control study. *J Natl Cancer Inst* 81:1560–1567, 1989.
18. Ziegler V: Chronic antigenic stimulation in the evolution of chronic dermatitis to lymphoma: an animal model? Presented at the European Contact Dermatitis Society meeting, Brussels, October 1992.
19. Lane CG, Rockwood EM, Sawyer CS, et al: Dermatoses of the hands. *JAMA* 128:987–993, 1945.
20. Rycroft RJG: Looking at work dermatologically. *Dermatol Clin* 6:1–5, 1988.
21. DeBoer EM, Bruynzeel DB, Van Ketel WG: Dyshidrotic eczema as an occupational dermatosis in metal workers. *Contact Dermatitis* 19:184–185, 1988.
22. Epstein E: Hand dermatitis: Practical management and current concepts. *J Am Acad Dermatol* 10:395–424, 1984.
23. Agrup G: Hand eczema and other hand dermatoses in South Sweden. *Acta Dermatol Venereol* 99:6–37, 1969.
24. Lammintausta K, Kalimo K, Havu VK: Occurrence of contact allergy and hand eczemas in hospital wet work. *Contact Dermatitis* 8:84–90, 1982.
25. Mathias CGT, Maibach HI: Cutaneous irritation: Factors influencing the response to irritants. *Clin Toxicol* 13:333–340, 1978.
26. Estlander T, Jolanski R: How to protect the hands. *Dermatol Clin* 6:105–114, 1988.
27. Berardinelli SP: Prevention of occupational skin disease through use of chemical protective gloves. *Dermatol Clin* 6:115–119, 1988.
28. Adams A: Patch testing: A recapitulation. *J Am Acad Dermatol* 5:637–651, 1981.
29. Rysted I: Factors influencing the occurrence of hand eczema in adults with a history of atopic dermatitis in childhood. *Contact Dermatitis* 12:185–195, 1985.
30. Sirot G: Nummular eczema. *Semin Dermatol* 2:68–74, 1983.
31. Menne T, Hjorth N: Pompholyx-dyshidrotic eczema. *Semin Dermatol* 2:57–59, 1983.
32. Meneghini CL, Angelini G: Contact and microbial allergy in pompholyx. *Contact Dermatitis* 5:45–50, 1979.
33. Schuppli R: Zur Atiologe der dyshidrosis. *Dermatologica* 108:393–398, 1954.
34. Kligman AM, Leyden JJ: Seborrheic dermatitis. *Semin Dermatol* 2:57–59, 1983.
35. Liden C: Contact allergy: A cause of facial dermatitis among visual display unit operators. *Am J Cont Dermatol* 1:171–176, 1990.
36. Fransway AF: Dermatoses in office workers. Presented at the Occupational Dermatology Symposium, meeting of the American Academy of Dermatology, 1991.
37. Fisher AA: A "Current Contact News" follow-up: Controversial subjects and those resulting in litigation. *Cutis* 52:254–256, 1993.
38. Jillson O: Dermatophytids. *Semin Dermatol* 2:68–74, 1983.
39. Stevenson CJ: Occupational vitiligo: Clinical and epidemiological aspects. *Br J Dermatol* 105:51–56, 1981.
40. Nordlund JJ: Vitiligo. In Thiers BH, Dobson RL (eds): *Pathogenesis of Skin Disease*. New York, Churchill Livingstone, 1986, pp 99–127.
41. Secretan H: Oedeme dur et hyperplasie traumatique du metacarpe dorsal. *Rev Med Suisse Romande* 21:409–415, 1911.

4

Patch Testing a Century Later

Christopher J. Gallant

Patch testing is a simple, direct biologic assay that can be used to identify and often confirm the cause of allergic contact dermatitis. It is without question the most important and often the only test used in the investigation of this common problem.

The patch test procedure has not changed much since it was described by Jadasson almost 100 years ago. He initially reported a patient who had developed a dermatitic reaction to mercury compounds after having used topical mercury plasters. Jadasson recognized the potential for dermatitic skin reactions to occur in some (sensitized) patients when chemicals were applied to their skin and thereby introduced the world to the contact test then referred to as *functionelle Hautprufung*.[1,2]

Refinement of the patch test as an investigative tool and its application to medical research are credited to Bruno Bloch, who originally studied with Jadasson.[3] It remained a relatively obscure and underutilized investigative tool until 1931, when Sulzberger and Wise presented a review of their work at the American Medical Association meeting. They introduced the test as we know it today to North America. Their report, published later that year, still serves as an important reference on the subject.[1]

Patch testing is a method by which a patient is reexposed, under controlled circumstances, to the chemical(s) thought to have caused the dermatitis. Although straightforward in design and simple in its premise, the patch test is not a perfect system. Successful use of this test is dependent upon careful patient selection, close attention to the standardized protocol for antigen application, and finally, critical interpretation of the test results.

Clinicians often equate a positive patch test with the fulfillment of Koch's postulate. They infer that because a patient with dermatitis has been shown to develop a positive reaction to compound X, that the same compound must therefore be the cause of the dermatitis. In utilizing the results of patch testing to make a diagnosis, a physician is extrapolating from an artificial test situation to real life and assuming that the results are valid under both sets of circumstances. Although in many cases this assumption is true, there are also clinical situations in which it could lead to erroneous conclusions. Interpretation of patch testing includes a determination both of the test result and of how relevant that result is to the patient's exposure. The patch test, whether positive or negative, is only one facet of this larger picture.

PATIENT SELECTION

The selection of suitable patients for patch testing is an important part of the process which is often overlooked. Some clinicians feel that patch testing should be used routinely on all patients being assessed for contact dermatitis. Others, Sulzberger included, suggest that the best results are obtained only if patients are carefully screened before testing.

The patch test is both sensitive (0.77) and specific (0.71), with a validity index of 0.74.[4] As with other sensitive medical tests, the number of false positives and false negatives increases and the predictive value of the test results drops if large numbers of low-risk patients are tested.[4] Furthermore, if large numbers of allergens are routinely used in a shotgun manner, the specificity of results also suffers.

In order to yield the best results, a thorough history followed by a careful clinical assessment must be completed on all patients prior to considering patch testing. This assessment not only ensures the best patient selection but also provides the detailed information essential for the accurate interpretation of test results.

TEST PROCEDURES AND MATERIALS

Bloch's original technique utilized a linen square soaked in the test chemical, occluded on normal skin (usually the back) with oiled silk, and fixed in place with adhesive plaster. He recommended leaving the materials in place for 24 hr and recorded observations at 24, 48, 72 hr and then again at intervals during the following 2 weeks.[1]

Today in most centers, the patch test materials are left in place for 48 hr. Readings are usually taken at 48 hr and 96 hr. A final reading at 1 week is also recommended. It has been demonstrated that a single reading at 48 hr will miss up to 34% of positive reactions.[5] Furthermore, if only the early reading is taken, false positives may result due to misinterpretation of irritant reactions which usually fade by the second reading. The late readings are most important for picking up delayed positive reactions to neomycin and some organic dyes which would otherwise be missed.[5]

Reactions appearing after 2 weeks usually mean that the patient has been sensitized to a test allergen by the patch test procedure itself. The latter is fortunately an uncommon occurrence when accepted test procedures are followed and the recommended test concentrations are used. The risk of inadvertently sensitizing a patient is greater when nonstandardized allergens are tested. It is important to discuss the potential risks and benefits of patch testing with each patient prior to testing.

There are some exceptions to the usual 48/96 hr schedule. These include tests where contact urticarial reactions may be involved and tests for clothing dermatitis.

Contact urticaria is a reaction pattern that has received little attention until recent years. It is interesting to review Sulzberger and Wise's recounting of Bloch's original description, in which he described, "a reaction in a patient so extremely hypersensitive that the patch had to be removed in 15 minutes."[1] This probably is one of the first clinical reports of contact urticaria. Fisher reports that there are at least four types of contact urticarial reactions that can be recognized; the most important of them, for this discussion, are nonallergic and allergic urticaria.[6]

There are some agents, including alcohol, benzoic acid, cinnamic acid, and balsam of Peru, that can cause contact urticaria in a large proportion of the nonsensitized general public. Reactions usually occur within 45 min and clear within 2 hr.

Allergic urticaria can also occur in patients who are sensitized to an antigen and have produced IgE antibodies. Foods are the most common allergens in this group. Others include proteins, antibiotics, and latex (natural rubber). This immediate response usually appears in the first 30 to 60 min after application. Tests with these allergens are often applied separately so that the patches can be examined without disturbing the other allergens. Patients in my office usually wait for 30 min before leaving the office after routine testing and at least 1 hr after testing for specific contact urticaria. They are asked to report intense itching immediately so that any urticarial responses can be identified. Contact urticaria is discussed in more detail in Chapter 7.

Patch tests for reactions to clothing or footwear often are negative if only 48 hr of contact with the material is used. Usually samples of the suspect clothing or footware are soaked for 10 to 15 min and then occluded on the skin for up to 5 days. This system results in a higher positive response rate.[7]

The patch test strips should be removed at least 10 min before the first reading is done. This allows the alternating pattern of blanching and erythema caused by pressure and the tape to fade. Dermatographism may appear in susceptible individuals and must be allowed to clear before the tests are read. Occasionally, occlusion can cause folliculitis or miliaria, which can be mistaken for positive reactions at the 48 hr reading. Delayed readings at 96 hr or later are essential if false positives and false negatives are to be avoided.

The most significant changes in patch testing have come in the form of improved test materials. There has been little change in the technique described above.

Tape

Adhesives used to hold the test materials on the skin have improved greatly. Formerly, tape reactions were quite common. Sulzberger and Wise, in the discussion of their paper, mused about the possible causes of tape reactions in some of their patients and suggested ways to avoid it.[1] Most systems currently use fine mesh paper tape with a polyacrylate adhesive which causes few reactions on the occluded skin.

Test Systems

A growing number of test systems are now available but most fall into one of three general categories.

First is the older Al-Test (IMECO, Stockholm) chambers, which were the standard for many years and are still in use. These consist of a filter paper disc attached to a plastic-coated foil strip (Figure 4-1). The materials to be tested were applied to the disc and then held in place on the skin by tape.

The Finn chamber (Epitest, Helsinki) is the most common example of the next group and consists of an aluminum or polypropylene disc about 8 mm in diameter fixed to a wide strip of Scanpor tape (Figure 4-1). It is generally considered the standard system and is used in most referral centers at this time. The Finn chamber system has streamlined the test process. It is more compact and simpler to apply. This allows more allergens to be tested at once. Rarely patients show contact allergy to the aluminum discs.[8]

The newest test systems consist of prepackaged kits that contain a selection of test allergens premeasured and already loaded on an adherent strip (Epiquick, Hermal, Germany; True test, *Pharmacia,* Sweden). Although the choice of allergens available in this format is limited at this time, both True test and Epiquick promise to increase the number in the near future. These systems seem to be the method of the future and may solve many of the standardization problems inherent in manually prepared systems. Extensive testing has shown that these systems produce reliable results comparable to those of conventional testing methods. The major drawbacks at this time are the limited number of available allergens and their cost.

TEST APPLICATION

Convention, standardization, and practicality dictate that most patch tests are applied on the back (Figure 4-2). When multiple panels of allergens are applied, there are few other sites where patches can be applied and not easily dislodged. It is essential that the allergens remain undisturbed in direct contact with the skin for the full 48 hr before being removed. Failure of the adhesive to hold is one of the most common causes of false-negative tests. To obtain the best possible results, test patches should be applied to dry, smooth skin with little hair. Some patients must be shaved before the patches are

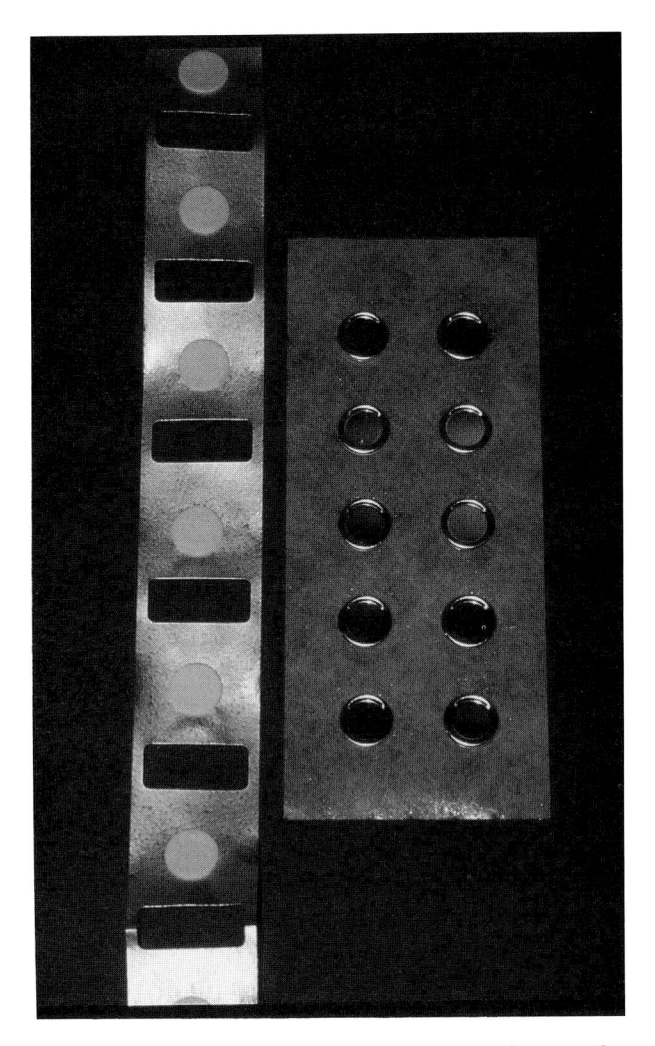

Figure 4-1. Al-Test strip (left), Finn chambers (right).

applied. If the skin is shaved, the patches should not be applied to abraded or inflamed skin. The flat area over the scapula provides a stable area with little movement. The midsection of the back over the spine should be avoided because movement will often dislodge the patches.

During the test period, the back must be kept dry and activities that might interfere with the patches should be avoided. If a portion of the patch loses contact with the skin, test results in that area are suspect and the tests should be repeated.

In addition to providing an easily accessible, large, stable site, the back is one of the most reactive sites for patch test reactions. Comparative testing has shown that there is a higher incidence of positive results on the upper back and forearms compared to the lower back, shins, hands, or feet.[9]

There are a few important situations in which areas other than the back

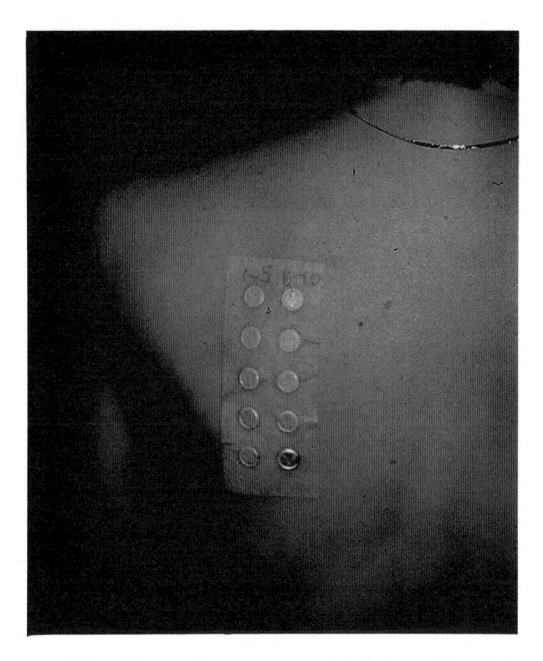

Figure 4-2. Finn chambers applied to patient's back.

should be used. One is in testing for contact reactions to food products, especially when an urticarial component is suspected. If possible, the affected site, usually the hand, should be used as the test site. It has been postulated that the larger antigenic proteins implicated in most food reactions only pass through already inflamed skin.

Another exception occurs when testing some allergens known to have particularly intense reactions that might scar, hyperpigment, or depigment the skin. Such allergens are usually tested on nonexposed, cosmetically less sensitive areas.

Gold can give persistent reactions and is therefore usually tested on the buttocks. Monobenzylether of hydroquinone and some irritants can cause depigmentation at test sites. These chemicals should obviously be used with caution by experienced clinicians and are also usually tested on the buttocks.

Once the patches are in place, it is often helpful to mark key reference points on the back with ink or fluorescent dye so that the test sites can be easily identified when the tapes are removed.

ALLERGENS

Allergens capable of eliciting an allergic contact reaction are generally small, simple chemicals that are usually less than 1000 daltons. Over 6 million substances are currently identified by their chemical structure; of these fewer than 3000 have been reported capable of sensitizing humans. One authoritative text provides reference information on 2800 allergens.[10]

TABLE 4-1 European Standard Tray*

1.	Potassium dichromate	0.5%
2.	p-Phenylenediamine	1%
3.	Thiuram mix	1%
4.	Neomycin sulfate	20%
5.	Cobalt chloride	1%
6.	Benzocaine	5%
7.	Nickel sulfate	5%
8.	Quinoline mix	6%
9.	Colophony	20%
10.	Paraben mix	15%
11.	Black rubber mix	0.6%
12.	Wool alcohols	30%
13.	Mercapto mix	2%
14.	Epoxy resin	1%
15.	Balsam of Peru	25%
16.	PTB formaldehyde resin	1%
17.	Mercaptobenzothiazole	2%
18.	Formaldehyde	1%
19.	Fragrance mix	8%
20.	Quaternium 15	1%
21.	Primin	0.01%
22.	Kathon CG	0.67%
23.	Sesquiterpene lactone	0.1%

*Available from Chemotechnique and Hermal (Europe).

The patient's history and physical examination will often strongly suggest the allergen responsible for the problem, thus narrowing the list of those that need to be tested. However, in many instances, no specific allergen is clearly responsible. In these cases, a screening tray (collection of allergens) is recommended.

Pooled data collected from patch testing centers around the world have identified a core group of about 100 allergens that account for most reactions. Several groups have further refined the data to develop a panel of about 25 allergens that represent the most common sensitizers implicated when the patient's history and physical examination fail to identify an obvious cause.[11] These collections are called *screening trays*. The ones most commonly used are the Hermal (United States) Allergen Patch Test Kit (see Table 1-2, p. 8) and the European Standard Tray. The contents of the European Standard Tray are listed in Table 4-1. Subtle differences in exposure and sensitization, between European and North American patients have resulted in minor variations in the allergens selected. Coordinated data collection and the use of computer-based data management quickly identify changes in population sensitivity patterns. Both groups regularly update these trays to reflect changes in allergen exposure and sensitization, as well as the introduction of new allergens into the marketplace. Periodically, the test concentrations of allergens and their vehicles are modified after analysis of pooled test results.

Specialized trays have been developed based on the unique exposures experienced by different occupational groups. Examples include dental, textile, and photography trays. Examples can be found in several texts (see Appendix 4-1 and Appendix 1).

Many chemicals can act as either allergens or irritants, depending on the concentration applied to the skin. Simple irritant responses are concentration dependent and can be standardized on non-sensitized subjects. To avoid false-positive irritant reactions, it is essential that only materials of known concentration, below the accepted irritant threshold, in a suitable base vehicle be used for patch testing.

It is unacceptable to patch test with unknown compounds or chemicals. These chemicals may cause injury to the patient, and the results are often uninterpretable due to irritation or contamination. It is rarely (if ever) acceptable to test industrial chemicals neat. Allergens should be carefully identified and test materials prepared as outlined in an appropriate reference. In the case of allergens for which reference material is not available, testing of standardized serial dilutions on a large number of test subjects is often needed to determine the test concentrations that reliably differentiate between irritant and allergic reactions. Whenever possible, allergens should be acquired from a reliable source such as those listed in Appendix 4-2 and Appendix 1.

Actual grading of test results takes experience. Practice and critical assessment of each reaction are essential to obtain reliable results. The current scoring system advocated by the North American Contact Dermatitis Group and the International Contact Dermatitis Groups is outlined in Table 4-2 (see also Figure 4-3).[12]

Although there is no reliable way to differentiate clinically between irritant and allergic reactions, there are patterns now generally recognized as suggestive of irritant reactions that are sometimes incorrectly interpreted as a positive patch test result.

Simple erythema without induration or vesiculation is usually a sign of irritation and has been commonly reported with potassium dichromate, wool

TABLE 4-2 Patch Test Scores

Test Score	Clinical Appearance	Abbreviation
1. Weak	Nonvesicular erythema, papules	+
2. Strong	Edematous, vesicular	+ +
3. Extreme	Bullous, ulcerative	+ + +
4. Doubtful	Erythema only	?
5. Irritant	Irritant reaction	R
6. Negative	No reaction	−
7. Excited skin	Multiple reactions	
8. Not tested		NT

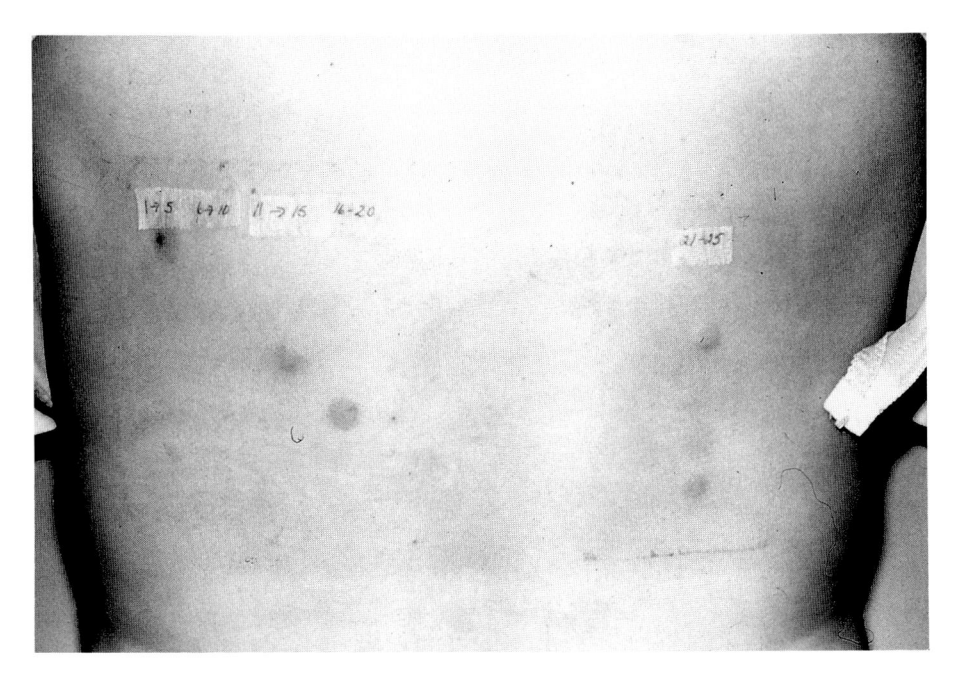

Figure 4-3. Multiple strong positive test reactions.

wax alcohols, formaldehyde, fragrance, and paraben mixes. The irritant erythema usually fades by the time of the second reading. Another sign of an irritant reaction is the so-called edge effect, in which there is a reaction at the edges of the test site but not at the center.[11] The repeated open application test (ROAT) is useful in determining the relevance of weak reactions to leave on consumer products.[12]

Pustular or follicular eruptions may also represent irritant reactions. Nickel, widely touted as the most common contact allergen, is also a potent irritant. The pustular irritant reaction caused by nickel is probably the most commonly reported false-positive patch test result.

Questionable weakly positive reactions should be repeated to try to confirm the response. In some situations, a serial dilution test is helpful in differentiating between irritant and questionable allergic responses. In rare situations, the test concentration of an allergen may need to be increased if false-negative reactions are suspected.

When used in the proper setting and by experienced physicians, the patch test has proved to be an invaluable tool. But as Sulzberger and Wise reported, there are many potential faults in this test system.[1] Sulzberger added to this list identifying other causes of false negatives (Table 4-3).[14]

Mitchell reported on the "angry back syndrome" in 1975. He noted that, in some cases, positive reactions seemed to appear in large groups, especially in patients who had developed an intense reaction to one or more of the test allergens.[15] Repeat testing of such patients revealed that up to 42% of the previously positive patches were negative when each patch was reapplied at separate visits.[16] Mitchell postulated that the presence of a strongly positive

TABLE 4-3 Common Causes of False Test Readings

False Positives	False Negatives
1. Irritant reactions	Too low test concentration
2. Dermatographism	Too little material applied
3. Angry back reaction	Poor contact with skin
4. Pressure reaction	Immunosuppressive drugs used
5. Contamination of allergens	Missed late reaction
6. Breakdown/separation of allergen preparation	
7. Occlusion effects	Test site less sensitive
8. Koebnerization of underlying dermatitis	Adjuvant factors missing (ie. friction, sweat, heat)
9.	Inappropriate test vehicle

response caused the surrounding skin to become "hyper-irritable," thus giving false-positive responses to other allergens.

Although the mechanism causing the irritable skin response has not been clearly documented, it is most likely very similar to the lowered irritant threshold identified in animals and humans with active sites of dermatitis or skin ulceration. The actual proportion of all test results that may be false positive is unknown but is less than 42% if patch testing is performed optimally.

The patch test does not exactly simulate the work environment in which some eruptions develop. It does not allow for potentially important interactions with physical factors or other chemicals in the work environment.

Changes in epidermal hydration due to increased humidity, occlusion or sweating may significantly alter transepidermal absorption, and thereby influencing cutaneous reactivity.

Exogenous factors such as heat and radiation may interact with either the allergen or the skin, thereby altering the cutaneous response. Ultraviolet radiation can influence both local and systemic immune responses and must therefore be considered a significant variable.[17]

INTERPRETATION OF RESULTS

A positive test result alone does not constitute a diagnosis of allergic contact dermatitis. Only if the patient or the investigator is able to relate the positive test result clearly to an exposure in the patient's environment that could plausibly be responsible for the clinical pattern of the dermatitis can the diagnosis be confirmed. It is just as common for patch test results to identify past allergens or apparently irrelevant positives. Experienced, well-read, and tenacious investigators are often able to link positive results to unexpected exposures.

Despite the widespread use of the patch test in the investigation of work-related skin disease, there is still some question about the relevance of a positive patch test in many situations. Patients frequently have positive patch tests to antigens not normally found in their environment. They may have persistent dermatitis despite withdrawal of the allergen suspected of causing their dermatitis or, conversely, may have resolution of the skin eruption despite continued exposure.

Ten percent or more of patients with no history of skin disease are found to have positive patch tests to allergens to which they were exposed.[18]

ADVERSE REACTIONS

As noted above, contact reactions may be intense and cause pigmentary changes and persistent irritation. In addition, distant sites of previous dermatitis or generalized ID reactions may occur when patients are reexposed to an allergen during testing.

Although the patch test is generally considered very safe, the potential for anaphylactic reactions has been well documented. Until recently type 1 immediate reactions were thought to be rare. However, they are commonly seen in patients sensitive to natural latex and some types of foods or antibiotics.[19] Since these same allergens are also well-documented causes of contact dermatitis and are included in patch testing, the potential for serious reactions is real. It behooves the clinician to be familiar with the properties of the allergens tested and to maintain a high level of suspicion if the patient's clinical history suggests anaphylactic type 1 responses. We now ensure that appropriate emergency equipment is available when testing is being conducted.

APPENDIX 4-1 Source Texts for Allergens and Specialized Allergen Trays

1. Adams RM: *Occupational Skin Disease.* Philadelphia, Saunders, 1990.
2. Cronin E: *Contact Dermatitis.* Edinburgh, Churchill-Livingstone, 1980.
3. Degroot AC: *Patch Testing Concentrations and Vehicles for 2800 Allergens.* Amsterdam, Elsevier, 1986.
4. Fisher AA: *Contact Dermatitis,* Rietschel RL, Fowler JE. (eds), 4 ed. Philadelphia, Lea & Febiger (in press).
5. Marks JG & DeLeo V: *Contact and Occupational Dermatology.* St. Louis, Mosby—Year Book, 1992.

APPENDIX 4-2 Patch Test Supply Sources

United States	Canada
Chemotechnique Diagnostics AB Products imported & distributed by: Dormer Labs will ship to the United States	Dormer Labs Inc. 91 Kelseid Unit 5 Rexdale, Ont M9W 5A3 Fax 416-242-9487 Phone 416-242-6167 1-800-363-5040
Trolabs Products imported & distributed by: Pharmascience will ship to the United States	Pharmascience (Omniderm) Inc. 8400 Darnley Rd., Montreal, Quebec H4T 1M4 Fax 514-342-7764 Phone 514-340-1114 1-800-363-8805

The Allergen Test Kit (Hermal, USA) is available directly from United States sources.
Hermal Pharmaceutical Labs Inc.
163 Delaware Ave,
Delmar, NY 12054
Phone 1-800-HERMAL-1
Fax 518-475-0180

REFERENCES

1. Sulzberger MB, Wise F. The contact or patch test in dermatology. *Arch Dermatol Syphol* 23:519–531, 1931.
2. Adams RM: Profiles of greats in contact dermatitis. *Am J Contact Dermatol* 4(1):58–59, 1993.
3. Adams RM, Fisher T: Diagnostic patch testing. In Adams *Occupational Skin Disease,* ed 2. Philadelphia, WB Saunders, 1990, p 223.
4. Nethercott JR, Holness DL: Validity of patch test screening trays. *J Am Acad Dermatol* 31(3):568, 1989.
5. Rietschel RL, Adams R, Maibach H, et al: The case for patch test readings beyond day 2. *J Am Acad Dermatol* 18(1):42–45, 1988.
6. Fisher AA: *Contact Dermatitis,* ed 3. Philadelphia, Lea & Febiger, 1986, p 686.
7. Fisher AA: *Contact Dermatitis,* ed 3. Philadelphia, Lea & Febiger, 1986, p 331.
8. Fisher AA: *Contact Dermatitis,* ed 3. Philadelphia, Lea & Febiger, 1986, p 854.
9. Magnusson B, Hersle K: Patch test methods. *Acta Dermatol* 45:257–261, 1965.
10. Degroot AC: *Patch Testing Concentrations and Vehicles for 2800 Allergens,* Amsterdam, Elsevier, 1986.

REFERENCES

11. Fischer T, Maibach H: Antigen preparation for the patch test. *Occup Med State of the Art Reviews* 1(2):343–348, 1986.
12. Adams RM: *Occupational Skin Disease*. Philadelphia, WB Saunders, 1990, pp 230–231.
13. Wahlberg JE: Use Tests in Contact Dermatitis. Rycroft RJG, Menné T, Frosh PJ, Benezra C. (eds). Berlin, Springer-Verlag, 1992, pp 261–262.
14. Sulzberger MB: The patch test—who should use it and why. *Contact Dermatitis* 1:117–119, 1975.
15. Mitchell JC: The angry back syndrome. *Contact Dermatitis* 1:193–194, 1975.
16. Bruynzeel DP, Maibach HI: Excited skin syndrome. *Arch Dermatol* 122:323–328, 1986.
17. Veien NK, Hattel T, Laurberg G: Is patch testing a less accurate tool in the summer months? *Amer J Contact Dermatitis* 3(1):35–36, 1992.
18. Magnusson B, Moller J: Contact allergy without skin disease. *Acta Derm Venereol* 59(85):113–115, 1979.
19. Fisher AA: *Contact Dermatitis,* ed 3. Philadelphia, Lea & Febiger, 1986.

5

Patch Testing Using Standard Screening Sets for Cases of Occupational Dermatitis

Elizabeth F. Sherertz

INTRODUCTION

Contact dermatitis is the most common occupational skin disease. Most occupational contact dermatitis (about 80%) is irritant, and the diagnosis is based on the history of exposures and appearance of the dermatitis. Approximately 20% of occupational contact dermatitis is allergic (ACD). Diagnosis of ACD is based on a history of exposure, clinical findings, and epicutaneous patch testing to document an allergy to an allergen. Interpretation of the relevance of the allergen to the workplace exposures and to the patient's dermatitis is important.

Dermatologists are sometimes discouraged from seeking a contact allergic factor for an eczematous dermatitis, particularly when the tedious question of work relatedness arises. There is a sense that the 20-item standard screening patch test tray available in the United States is inadequate for the evaluation of occupational ACD, and patients may go undiagnosed if patch testing is not done for this reason.[1] Experience with patch testing of patients indicates that the standard screening series (Table 5-1) unveils about 80% of the relevant contact allergy for the general public but may detect only about 50% of occupational ACD.[2] This does not include poison oak/poison ivy ACD, which is an important cause of occupational ACD[3] but one that is rarely included in patch test series since a large percentage of those exposed are presumed to be allergic to poison ivy/oak.

In this chapter, the usefulness of the standard screening series of allergens is reviewed as a starting point in the evaluation of occupational ACD. The use of occupation-specific or allergen-specific screening trays is also considered.

THE STANDARD SCREENING SERIES

In the United States, a series of 20 allergens is currently available for patch test use (Table 5-1). This series is variably called the *standard tray*, the *AAD tray* (although the American Academy of Dermatology no longer markets it), or the *North American tray* (referring to the standard screening allergens used by physicians in the United States and Canada or to the series suggested for screening by the North American Contact Dermatitis Group). The European standard (see Table 4-1, p 47) series is often mentioned in the literature and contains most of the same allergens, with the addition of cobalt chloride, quinoline mix, paraben mix, fragrance mix, sesquiterpene lactone mix, and 5-chloro-2-methyl-4-isothiazolin 3-one and 2-methyl-4-isothiazolin 3-one and the deletion of cinnamic aldehyde, carba mix, ethylenediamine, and imidazolidinyl urea. Let us briefly review the standard allergens, and some of the occupational sources of exposure to each.

Rubber Allergens

Mercaptobenzothiazole, carba mix, thiuram mix, mercapto mix, and black rubber mix are standard allergens mostly related to rubber products. Thus, detection of rubber allergy represents 20% of the screening series. Contact urticaria to rubber latex cannot be diagnosed using these patch test allergens.

Mercaptobenzothiazole (MBT)

MBT is a rubber accelerator used to speed up the vulcanization process. MBT also has many nonrubber uses, especially as an additive in cutting oils, anticorrosive agents, cements, adhesives, industrial greases, film emulsions, veterinary flea products, and fungicides. The most common source of exposure leading to sensitization is rubber, particularly in footwear or gloves.

Case example. A 43-year-old woman had a long history of foot dermatitis that improved when she wore nonrubber shoes. She started working in a factory producing machinery parts and within 2 months developed vesicular hand dermatitis. Patch tests demonstrated a positive reaction to MBT, which was felt to be relevant to both her footwear dermatitis and her hand dermatitis. The latter may be considered a work-related exacerbation of a preexisting

TABLE 5-1 Standard Screening Patch Test Allergens* and Occupational Sources†

Allergen/Concentration	Other Names	Occupational Source Examples
Rubber Allergens		
Mercaptobenzothiazole, 1% pet‡	MBT 2-benzathiazalethiol	Rubber shoes or insoles, gloves Rubber manufacture Anticorrosion agents Rubber parts, devices Cutting oils, greases Veterinary products
Carba Mix, 3% pet 1,3-Diphenylguanidine (1%) Zinc diethyldithiocarbamate (1%) Zinc dibutyldithiocarbamate (1%)	DPG, ZBC, ZDC	Rubber gloves, shoes, insoles Agricultural fungicides/insecticides Rubber manufacture
Thiuram mix, 1% pet Tetramethyl thiuram disulfide (.25%) Tetramethyl thiuram monosulfide (.25%) Tetraethyl thiuram disulfide (.25%) Dipentamethylene thiuram disulfide (.25%)	TMTD, TETD, TMTM, PTH Thiuram	Rubber gloves, masks Medical devices Rubber manufacture Agricultural fungicides/insecticides
Black rubber p-Phenylenediamine mix, 0.6% pet N-phenyl-N-cyclohexyl-p-phenylenediamine (0.25%) N-isopropyl-N-phenyl-p-phenylenediamine (0.1%) N-diphenyl-p-phenylenediamine (0.25%)	CPPP, IPPD, DPPD	Tires, black rubber tubing, gaskets, parts Black rubber boots, gloves, masks Rubber manufacture
Mercapto mix, 1% pet N-cyclohexyl-2-benzothiazole-sulfonamide (0.333%) 2,2-Benzothiazyl disulfide (0.333%) 4-Morpholinyl-2-benzothiazyl disulfide (0.333%)	CBS, MBTS, MMBT	Rubber manufacture Rubber gloves, shoes, insoles Agricultural repellents, disinfectants Photographic film emulsion Cutting oils

56

Metal Allergens

Nickel sulfate, 2.5% pet
- Metal tools, instruments, parts
- Batteries
- Metal-cutting fluids, coolants
- Ceramics manufacture
- Metal plating

Potassium dichromate, 0.25% pet
- Chromium
- Chrome
- Chromate
- Cement
- Tanned leather work boots
- Textile dyes, prints
- Automotive manufacturing
- Electroplating, welding
- Ceramics
- Brick foundries
- Blueprints
- Metal alloy production
- Inks
- Milk testing

Adhesive/Plastics

Colophony, 20% pet
- Rosin
- Qum rosin
- Tall oil
- Abietic acid, alcohol
- Baseball, violin rosin
- Paper
- Printing inks
- Solder flux
- Adhesive
- Varnish, coatings
- Dental impression paste
- Pine cleaners

Epoxy resin, 1% pet
- 4, 4-Isopropylidene Diphenol-epichlorhydrin
- Diglycidyl ether
- Bisphenol A
- Epichlorhydrin
- Adhesives
- Laminates
- Paints, inks, polyvinyl chloride
- Electrical coatings
- Vinyl gloves

p-Tert-butylphenol formaldehyde, 1% pet
- PTBP formaldehyde
- 4 (1, 1-Dimethylethyl) phenol
- Adhesive for leather, cardboard, plywood
- Dental bonding

TABLE 5-1 (Continued)

Allergen/Concentration	Other Names	Occupational Source Examples
Biocides/Preservatives		
Formaldehyde, 1% aqueous	Methanal	Disinfectants
	Formalin	Leather tanning
		Urea and phenolic resins
		Paper manufacture
		Metal working fluids
		Particle board
		Textile finishes
		Fixative, embalming
		Hand lotion, soaps
Quaternium 15, 2% pet	N-(3-chloroallyl) hexaminium chloride	Metal working fluids
	Dowicil 200	Latex paints, paperboard
	Methanamine-3-chloroallylochloride	May cross-react with formaldehyde
		Jointing cements or adhesives
Imidazolidinyl urea, 2% aqueous	N,N-methylenebis (N-)1-(hydroxymethyl)	Hand lotion, topical creams
	2,5-Dioxo-4-imidazolidinyl urea	May cross-react with formaldehyde
	Germall 115	
Medications		
Benzocaine, 5% pet	Ethyl aminobenzoate	First aid/employee clinic
	p-Aminobenzoic acid ethyl ester	First aid/burn spray-creams
		Cough drops, sore throat lozenges
		Topical pain relievers
		PABA-containing sunscreen
Neomycin sulfate, 20% pet		Topical antibiotic drops, spray, ointments

Fragrance/Flavoring
Cinnamic aldehyde, 1% pet   Cinnamal   Manufacture of fragranced or
                             3-Phenyl-2-propenal   flavored products
                                                         Bakery spices, flavorings exposure

Balsam of Peru, 25% pet   Balsam   Manufacture of fragranced or
                             Benzylbenzoate   flavored products
                             Benzylcinnamate   Bakery spices, flavorings exposure

Miscellaneous
Lanolin alcohol, 30% pet   Wool wax alcohol   Hand cleaners
                             Anhydrous lanolin   Polishes, waxes
                                                          Corrosion preventative
                                                          Cutting oil emulsions

p-phenylenediamine, 1% pet   PPD   Hairdresser dyes
                             1, 4-Benzenediamine   Azo textile dye production
                             1, 4-Phenylenediamine   Photographic developers
                             p-Diaminobenzene   Rubber manufacture
                                                          Inks
                                                          Oils, greases

Ethylenediamine dihydrochloride, 1% pet   1, 2-Ethanediamine   Emulsifiers
                                          1, 2-Diaminoethane   Epoxy and textile resin hardeners
                                          Chlor-ethanmine   Color developers
                                                                Solvents for shellac, albumin
                                                                Electroplating gels

---

*Standard allergens from Hermal Pharmaceutical Laboratories, Inc., Delmar, NY.
†Examples of possible occupational exposure: history and determination of patient-specific exposure is important. Consult contact dermatitis texts.[4,13–15]
‡pet = petrolatum.

59

condition, as the triggering exposures to industrial rubber gloves and to machinery oil containing MBT as a corrosion inhibitor were unique to her workplace exposure. Modification of her job duties led to improvement in her dermatitis.

Mercapto Mix

This mixture of thiazole accelerators (Table 5-1) has an exposure list similar to that of MBT, mainly associated with natural or synthetic rubber products.

Thiuram Mix

This mix consists of four chemicals (Table 5-1) used as rubber accelerators. Nonrubber sources include some germicides, insecticides and antiseptics, adhesives, paints, and shampoos/soaps. One of the thiurams, tetramethylthiuram disulfide, is used systematically as disulfiram (Antabuse) for the treatment of alcohol abuse. Thiuram is currently the most frequent allergen identified in cases of ACD to rubber sensitivity products.[5] Most cases of sensitivity to thiuram are due to rubber gloves. This is an increasingly frequent problem in the health care industry and parallels the recommendation of "universal precautions," which has led to more rapid manufacture of gloves and more frequent use. Unfortunately, "hypoallergenic" gloves are usually not the answer to ACD to rubber gloves.[6] Patch testing to confirm an allergy to thiuram or other rubber allergens and appropriate selection of glove alternatives are essential for clinical improvement[7] (see Appendix 4. p 160).

Carba Mix

(Table 5-1). These agents are used as rubber accelerators, as fungicides, and in the manufacture of plastics. There is controversy as to whether the carbamates are necessary on the screening series, since there is cross-reactivity with the thiurams, so that both may be positive 85% of the time.[8,9] When carba reacts alone, it is more likely to be due to the diphenylguanidine portion, and its typical exposure sources are industrial tubing or hoses.

Black Rubber Mix

This is a mixture of *p*-phenylenediamines, as outlined in Table 5-1. These are used as antioxidants in rubber manufacture and, because of their color, are used mainly in gray or black rubber; hence, they are more likely to be found in industrial or automotive use. A common sensitizing exposure is vehicle tires. Patients reacting to black rubber mix should have a thorough evaluation for an occupational exposure, as consumer rubber products in prolonged contact with the skin are less likely to have these phenylenediamines.

Metal Allergens

Nickel

The standard series has nickel and potassium dichromate as the metal allergens. Nickel is an extremely common allergen, and initial sensitization may occur with personal products such as pierced earrings or clothing snaps. Sensitized patients can subsequently be exposed to nickel-plated products in the workplace and develop dermatitis at sites not previously involved (e.g., the hands). If this occurs, it is important to try to minimize workplace exposure, either by using protective clothing (appropriate gloves, sleeves over machinery) or by changing to stainless steel or nickel-free instruments (e.g., hairdresser scissors). The dimethylglyoxime test kit (see Chapter 10) for nickel detection is useful to take into the workplace to narrow the list of which metal materials contain nickel.

Case Example. A 33-year-old woman without pierced ears developed a vesicular hand dermatitis in August 3 months after beginning work with a landscaping maintenance business. A careful history revealed that the problem became worse after she increased the hand watering of plants using a metal hand-held spray nozzle, which she switched from one hand to the other. The history and patch testing ruled out other allergens. A positive patch test to nickel and a positive dimethylglyoxime test of the spray nozzle implicated it as a causative factor for the woman's work-related dermatitis. Substitution of a plastic spray device greatly improved her dermatitis, which was slow to heal because of irritant exposures.

Potassium Dichromate

Chromate allergy can cause a debilitating chronic contact dermatitis that is difficult to clear even if the exposure is removed. Earlier detection of a chromate allergy, through suspicion and patch testing, does improve the prognosis.[10] The main source of occupational exposure to chromates is from cement.[11]

A secondary occupational source of chromate is from chromate-tanned leather in work boots, utility belts, or leather gloves. It is expensive and difficult to obtain chromate-free work boots, but this may be necessary to keep an employee on the job.

Preservatives/Biocides

The standard allergen panel has the following preservatives: formaldehyde, quaternium 15, and imidazolidinyl urea. These are found in many skin care products, creams, lotions, and liquid soaps. Formaldehyde is a base component of a number of industrial processes, examples of which are given in Table 5-2. Further, these preservatives (biocides) have different names in the industrial setting than those used in the standard tray (Table 5-3). Biocides are incorpo-

TABLE 5-2 Formaldehyde Uses in Industry

Agriculture—disinfectants
Auto mechanics—metal and tire cleaners
Baking—disinfectants and cleaners
Beauticians/cosmetologists—cosmetic products
Cleaning/housekeeping—cleansers and disinfectants
Construction—solvents, adhesives, and glues
Dental/medical/veterinary—disinfectants and medications
Dry cleaning—spot removers
Electronics—metal cleaners
Embalmers—formalin
Laboratory/pathology—formalin
Machinists—biocides in cutting fluids
Metal working—metal cleaners
Painting/paper hanging—resins in paints and wallpapers
Paper manufacture—formaldehyde and resins
Particleboard/plywood manufacture—formaldehyde resins
Pest control—disinfectants
Photography—developers
Printing—inks
Textile working—fabric finishes

Source: Adapted from Feinman SE: *Formaldehyde Sensitivity and Toxicity.* Boca Raton, FL, CRC Press, 1988.

rated into water-based cutting fluids, coolants, water baths, and heating and air-conditioning systems. Several biocides are based on the release of formaldehyde, including quaternium 15 and imidazolidinyl urea (Table 5-3), but formaldehyde may not be an adequate screening allergen for these biocides. When possible, appropriate dilutions of the specific biocide should be tested.

Adhesives/Plastics

The standard allergen series has colophony (rosin), epoxy, and *p*-tert-butylphenol formaldehyde resin, which are primarily associated with adhesive or plastic systems, though other occupational sources are noted in Table 5-1.

Colophony

Colophony (rosin) is used in soldering flux, paper and printing inks, and as a tackifier in coatings, varnishes, and glues. It cross-reacts with turpentine spirits.

TABLE 5-3 Biocides (Antimicrobials, Preservatives)

Standard Series
  Formaldehyde*
  Imidazolidinyl urea*
  Quaternium 15*
Others
  1,2-Benzoisothiazolin-3-one
  Benzyl alcohol, chlorhexidine digluconate
  Benzyl salicylate
  2-Bromo-2-nitropropane-1, 3-diol*
  Butyl hydroxytoluene (BHT)
  Butyl hydroxyanisole (BHA)
  Chloracetamide
  1- (3-Chloroallyl)-3, 4, 7-triaza-1-azonia adamantine chloride*
  Chloramine-T
  Chlorocresol
  2-Chloro-N (hydroxymethyl) acetamide*
  2-Chloro-N-hydroxymethylacetamide
  Chloroxylenol
  Chlorquinaldol
  Clioquinol
  Diazolidinyl urea*
  DM DM Hydantoin*
  Glutaraldehyde
  Hexahydro-1, 3, 5-triethyl-5-triazine*
  Hexahydro-1, 3, 5-tris (2-hydroxyethyl)-5-triazine*
  Hexahydro-3, 5-tris (2-hydroxyethyl)-5-triazine*
  Hexylresorcinol
  Hydroxybenzoates
  2(2-Hydroxy-5-methyl phenyl) benzotriazole
  Methylchloroisothiazolinone/methylisothiazolinone
  2-n-Ocytyl-4-isothiazolin-3-one
  Parabens
  Phenoxyethanol
  Phenylmercuric acetate
  Phenylmercuric nitrate
  Sorbic acid
  Thiomersal
  Triclosan
  Tris
  1, 3, 5-Tris (2-hydroxyethyl)-hexahydrotriazine
  Tris (hydroxymethyl) nitromethane*

*Formaldehyde-releasing product.

Uncured Epoxy Resin

Epoxy resin allergy often results from exposure to two-component adhesive systems. It is also a problem in industries such as electrical and other parts assembly, aircraft maintenance, paint manufacture, and laminate or plastics manufacture.

Case Example. A 28-year-old man had a 4-month history of a vesicular hand dermatitis with patchy spread on his forearms, neck, and face. The dermatitis improved during a 1-week vacation from work. For 2 years he had worked in the manufacture of custom golf clubs, where part of the job required gluing the golf grip to the club using a two-part epoxy-based adhesive. Airborne contact dermatitis to epoxy was confirmed based on this exposure (with other sources of uncured epoxy exposure ruled out) and a positive patch test to epoxy resin from the standard tray. Moving to a well-ventilated area of the workplace and working away from the epoxy materials allowed this man to continue his work without recurrence of the dermatitis.

p-*Tert-Butylphenol Formaldehyde Resin*

This is used primarily as an adhesive for flexible synthetic or rubber components such as those used in shoes, watchbands, belts, boxes, and handbags. It is also used in household woodworking or ceramics glues, so nonoccupational exposures should be ruled out.

Topical Medications

Occupational skin injuries are much more common than dermatitis. On-the-job first-aid measures can lead to severe ACD which clinically resembles an eczematous reaction and a nonhealing injury. Benzocaine-containing anesthetic first-aid preparations and neomycin-containing antibiotics are important sources of potential contact allergy to topical medications. Workplace exposure to these elements as a source of the dermatitis should be ruled out.

Benzocaine

In addition to benzocaine's use as a first-aid preparation, industrial exposure to cross-reacting chemicals of benzoic acid derivatives should be ruled out. Examples include para-aminobenzoic acid (PABA), pharmaceutical manufacture or medical exposure to sulfonamides, and *p*-phenylenediamine dyes.

Neomycin

By far the most likely occupational exposure to neomycin is from first-aid topical antibiotic treatments. It may occasionally be found in veterinary preparations.

Fragrances/Flavorings

There are thousands of individual fragrance ingredients, and the screening series has two allergens that relate to fragrance sensitivity. Although personal products are most often implicated when a person has fragrance allergy, it is striking to think of the many possible occupational sources of fragrance, from additives to machinery oils and air conditioners, to air freshener, to cosmetic manufacture and sales, to tobacco flavoring, to patient care.

Cinnamic Aldehyde

Workers exposed to cinnamon spice substitutes may develop allergic reactions to cinnamic aldehyde. Handling some plants (e.g., hyacinth) or plant-derived oils (e.g., cassia oil) may be a problem. Maintenance personnel who handle strongly scented cleaners may also be at risk.

Balsam of Peru

This naturally occurring mixture of resins is used in pharmaceutical products, as well as in fragrances and flavorings. Bakers who handle spices may develop reactions to this product. Cross-reactions may occur with colophony, turpentine, and wood tars.

Miscellaneous Sources

p-Phenylenediamine

This black dye is used for permanent and semipermanent hair dye, so hairdressers may develop allergy to this substance, usually manifesting as hand dermatitis. Other sources of occupational exposure are printing/lithography inks, oils, greases, photocopying or photographic developers, and products used the production of azo textile dyes or in the rubber industry.

Lanolin (Wool Alcohol)

A major worksite source of lanolin is hand cleaners, hand lotions, and soaps. It may also be found in furniture polishes, waxes, corrosion inhibitors, cutting oils, paper, inks, textiles, and fur.

Ethylenediamine Dihydrochloride

There are numerous uses of ethylenediamine in industry, particularly as a hardener in epoxy resin systems. It may also be found in some solvents, and it is used as an emulsifier in topical creams. It may be a component of electroplating gels and color developers, and it is used for textile resins and lubricants. In general, ethylenediamine tetraacetic acid (EDTA) does not cross-react in patients allergic to ethylenediamine dihydrochloride.

FINDING THE STANDARD ALLERGEN IN THE WORKPLACE

Once a positive reaction to a standard allergen is found, it is important to look at workplace, home, hobby, and second-job exposures. Having the physician and patient go over possible exposures together is more useful than handing a textbook list to a patient or instructing the patient to simply read labels or Material Safety Data Sheets. Employee, employers, other health care providers, and the physician must understand the following:

1. Slow or minimal improvement away from the work site does not exclude work as a potential source of exposure.
2. Material Safety Data Sheets do not list all ingredients. Sometimes ingredients that are not hazardous or that are present in amounts of less than 1% in the material may cause contact allergy but may not be listed on the label.
3. Contact allergy may develop even after months or years of exposure. There does not have to be something new in the workplace.
4. Dermatitis appearing at a new site, or exacerbation of preexisting dermatitis due to workplace exposure to an allergen, also may be considered a work-related problem.[12]
5. Negative reactions to the standard screening patch test series do not totally rule out the possibility of ACD. If clinical suspicion remains strong, additional patch testing with appropriate substances may be indicated.

Case Example. A 26-year-old hairdresser had reported mild chapping of the hands since beginning his career several years previously. In the last 3 months, however, the eruption had become dramatically worse, with painful and itching blisters of the finger tips, which led to cracking and time missed from work. Rubber gloves did not seem to help. Patch tests with the standard series were negative. Additional patch tests with a "hairdressing series" (see Appendix 1) showed a positive patch test to glyceryl thioglycolate, which is found in acid permanent wave solutions. Avoidance of those permanent wave products, and of cutting the hair of clients who had those permanents, led to gradual improvement of his hand dermatitis to an acceptable and controllable baseline.

ALLERGEN SERIES FOR SPECIFIC OCCUPATIONS

Textbooks such as *Adams' Occupational Skin Disease*[13] or those by Fisher,[14] Rycroft et al.,[15] and Marks and DeLeo[4] present information about potential exposures to irritants and allergens in specific work settings ranging from agriculture to wine making. Adams devotes a large portion of his book to suggested allergens to test as supplements to the standard series. He has also presented some allergen lists in the dermatologic literature for occupational groups frequently at risk, such as cosmetologists/hairdressers, machinists, and dentists.[16] (See also Table 5-4.)

TABLE 5-4 Occupations at Higher Risk for Allergic Contact Dermatitis

Agriculture and forestry	Manufacturing
Construction	Assembly of parts
Dental and medical	Ceramics
Food and plant handling	Electronics
Hairdressing	Furniture
Housekeeping/maintenance	Textiles
Machinist	Photography
	Printing

Source: Adapted from Ref. 4.

TABLE 5-5 Other Occupation-Specific Trays,* with Examples of Allergens Missed by Standard Tray Screening

Bakery Series
 Benzoic acid
 Benzoyl peroxide
Dental Series
 Methyl methacrylate
 Ethylene glycol dimethacrylate
 Other acrylates
 Eugenol
Hairdressing Series
 Glyceryl monothioglycolate
 Resorcinol
Oil and Cutting Fluid Series
 1, 2-Benzisothiazolin-3-one
 2-Bromo-2-nitropropane-1, 3-diol
 4-Chloro-3-cresol
 4-Chloro-3-xylenol (PCMX)
 Hydrazine sulfate
 Methylchloroisothiazolinone
 Triethanolamine
Plastic/Adhesive/Isocyanate Series
 Bisphenol A
 Dibutyl phthalate
 Ethyl acrylate
   Other acrylates
 Hexamethylenetetramine
 2-n-Octyl-4-isothiazolin-3-one
 Phenyl glycidyl ether
 Toluene diisocyanate
   Other diisocyanates
 Tricresylphosphate
 Triethylenetetramine
 Triglycidyl isocyanurate

Photographic Series
 4-amino-N, N-diethylaniline sulfate
 Color developers
 Hydroxylammonium chloride
Rubber Additive Series
 Diphenylguanidine
 Diaminodiphenylmethane
 Diethylthiourea
   Other thioureas
Textile Colors and Finish Series
 Disperse dyes
 Dimethylol dihydroxyethylene urea
 Ethylene urea, melamine formaldehyde
Urea formaldehyde

*Consult companies for specific tray substances available (see Appendix 1).
 Trolabs   Chemotechnique Diagnostics AB
 Omniderm, Inc.   Dormer Laboratories
 8400 Darnley Road   6600 TransCanada Highway
 Montreal, Quebec, Canada   Pointe-Claire, Quebec, Canada
 514-340-1114   514-697-0519.

Chemotechnique and Hermal, European companies that manufacture patch test allergens, also have allergen panels designed for specific occupations (see Appendix 1). Such panels should be used to supplement, not replace, the use of the standard series (Table 5-5). If a physician works frequently with patients in specific occupational settings, it is worthwhile to have available additional patch test allergens targeted for those settings, or to refer patients in whom ACD is suspected but the standard screening series is negative to a dermatologist who has more specific allergens available.

SUMMARY

It is valuable to use the standard screening patch test allergen sets for the intended use of attempting to confirm suspected allergic contact dermatitis. Taking the time to understand workplace exposures and to interpret the relevance of the positive patch tests to these exposures and for the patient's dermatitis is important and rewarding. Office dermatologists should begin the investigation of occupational contact dermatitis using readily available standard patch test supplies.

REFERENCES

1. James WD, Rosenthal LE, Brancaccio RR, et al: American Academy of Dermatology Patch testing survey: Use and effectiveness of this procedure. *J Am Acad Dermatol* 26:991–994, 1992.
2. Menné T, Dooms-Goossens A, Wahlberg JG, et al: How large a proportion of contact sensitivities are diagnosed with the European standard series? *Contact Dermatol* 26:201–202, 1992.
3. Epstein WL: Poison oak and poison ivy dermatitis as an occupational problem. *Cutis* 13:544–548, 1974.
4. Marks JG Jr, DeLeo VA: *Contact and Occupational Dermatology.* St Louis, Mosby Year Book, 1992.
5. von Hintzenstern J, Hesse J, Koch HV, et al: Frequency, spectrum, and occupational relevance of type IV allergies to rubber chemicals. *Contact Dermatol* 24:244–252, 1991.
6. Hamann CP: Natural rubber latex protein sensitivity in review. *Am J Contact Dermatol* 4:4–21, 1993.
7. Rich P, Belozer ML, Norris P, et al: Allergic contact dermatitis to two antioxidants in latex gloves: 4, 4-thiobis (6-tert-butyl-meta-cresol) (Lowinox 44536) and butylhydroxyanisole. *J Am Acad Dermatol* 24:37–43, 1991.
8. Rademaker M, Forsyth A: Carba mix: A useful indication of rubber sensitivity. In Frosch PJ, Dooms-Goossens A, Lachapelle J-M (eds): *Current Topics in Contact Dermatitis.* New York, Springer-Verlag, 1989, pp 136–139.
9. Andersen KE, Burrows D, Cronin E, et al: Recommended charges to standard series. *Contact Dermatol* 19:389–390, 1988.

REFERENCES

10. Halbert AR, Gebauer KA, Wall LM: Prognosis of occupational chromate dermatitis. *Contact Dermatol* 27:214–219, 1992.
11. Bruze M, Fregert S, Gruvberger B: Patch testing with cement containing iron sulfate. *Dermatol Clin* 8:173–176, 1990.
12. Mathias CGT: Contact dermatitis and workers' compensation criteria for establishing occupational causation and aggravation. *J Am Acad Dermatol* 20:842–848, 1989.
13. Adams RM (ed): *Occupational Skin Disease,* ed 2. Philadelphia, WB Saunders, 1990.
14. Fisher AA: *Contact Dermatitis,* ed 3. Philadelphia, Lea & Febiger, 1986.
15. Rycroft RJG, Menné T, Frosch PJ, et al (eds): *Textbook of Contact Dermatitis.* New York, Springer-Verlag, 1992.
16. Adams RM: Panels of allergens for specific occupations. *J Am Acad Dermatol* 21:869–874, 1989.

6

Patch Testing to Allergens Not Found in the Standard Trays

Arthur D. Daily

This chapter is mandated by the numerous patients who come into the office with containers of things that they believe are causing their dermatitis. This is especially true of industry-related contact dermatitis. In the scope of one chapter, it is not possible to cover completely what to do and how to patch-test all of these patients. Instead, I present practical guidelines for patch testing in some of the more common occupational settings. For specific patch testing to volatile and irritant industrial and occupational chemicals, the reader is referred to the excellent textbooks[1-3] covering this subject.

    I have chosen to present this material in a manner which covers groups of occupational contact rather than specific chemical exposure. The reason is quite simple: Patients usually bring in products in which either the contents are not labeled or the ingredients are numerous and varied. Obviously, patch testing to such raw materials is no substitute for patch testing to the well-established, standardized antigens that are available. Testing to established antigens not only allows more specific identification but also avoids the pitfalls that often accompany "as is" testing. The most common of these pitfalls is the attempt to differentiate irritant from allergic reactions; even the best patch testers agree on the difficulty of making this distinction. On the other hand, there are occasions when dermatologists would miss the etiologic agent if they relied solely on standardized antigens. Further, in many situations, as-is testing provides reliable, positive information (e.g., plants, cosmetics, and over-the-counter [OTC] medications). Also, as we gain new and reliable information regarding contact urticaria, it becomes increasingly important to perform such testing. The entire issue of reactions to latex glove and latex rubber devices used in the health care industry is a prime example of contact urticaria. Some of these reactions are extremely serious—even life-threatening. Lastly, I encourage researching briefly raw materials in standard texts[4-8] to avoid certain predictable, irritant, or false-positive or -negative reactions.

HEALTH CARE WORKERS

The chemicals to which doctors, nurses, dentists, and associated hospital and laboratory personnel are exposed number in the hundreds. Some of the earliest descriptions of allergic contact dermatitis were reported to topically applied antibiotics; this condition was seen not only in patients but also in health care workers who applied them. Today the number of allergens is greatly expanded although allergy to neomycin and merthiolate (Thimersal) remain two of the most common, severe reactions encountered. This is partly due to their incorporation in a variety of OTC topical preparations. Very recently, Gentimycin has been demonstrated to be the most potent sensitizer among topical antibiotics. A more subtle exposure occurs through the handling of liquid medications, capsules, and pills by nurses; some of the earliest reactions to Thorazine were identified by this type of exposure.

Among this wide variety of topical agents used by physicians and other health care workers, the majority can be tested as is, using the 48-hr occlusion technique. In testing some of the germicides and disinfectants used in hospitals and physicians'/dentists' offices, dilution is required; this is often outlined in the Material Safety Data Sheet (MSDS) for the product. As a rule, testing to 0.1% and 1% solutions in a suitable vehicle is appropriate. With regard to pills, capsules, and liquid medications, Fisher's "Blue Pages" provides suggested concentrations and vehicles for patch testing.[4]

There are a few areas of contact dermatitis in which as-is testing presents unique problems. The most prevalent of these is reactions to the myriad natural latex rubber equipment used in the health care industry. Most of these reactions are type I reactions and thus require innovative testing techniques. Since anaphylactic reactions have occurred, with death in some patients, the sensitivity level is extreme in some cases. Testing often involves cutting up some of the raw latex product, extraction in a small volume of water, and then prick-testing, utilizing the forearm. Control testing, utilizing histamine and saline, should be done at the same time; because of the severity of some reactions, epinephrine and resuscitative equipment should be available. This subject has been covered in recent articles,[9,10] and dermatologists should bring themselves up-to-date on this important topic (see Chapter 7).

A second special area is that of contact dermatitis to acrylic and cyanoacrylate glues, such as those used in orthopedic bone cements, in dental appliances, and as adhesives in certain other related medical procedures. These substances are highly volatile and can even penetrate standard operating gloves. The degree of sensitivity and the variety of severe hand dermatitis that can develop as a result of exposure to these chemicals makes them unique. As of this writing, most of these substances can be patch-tested as is in the dried (cured) form; however, most allergens are now available in standardized patch test concentrations.[11,12]

Lastly, it is my premise that many cases of allergic contact dermatitis in health care workers are overlooked. It is imperative that one have a high index of suspicion and an open mind. In almost any contact situation—both airborne and direct—the vast majority of such contact sources can be tested as is, and taking a thorough history is the essential ingredient in guiding one to the likely sources of antigens.

FOOD HANDLERS, CHEFS, AND GOURMET COOKS

On a day-to-day basis, new restaurants are opening and many private citizens are taking to the kitchen in pursuit of a healthier, more tasty diet. Along with this burgeoning industry comes contact with a variety of foods, spices, and other accoutrements, as well as the metal, plastic, and wood devices required to mix and stir. Contact dermatitis, both urticarial and eczematous, is well known and has been described for many of these contactants. On the other hand, many are overlooked, and the use of standard screening trays is insufficient to uncover the wide variety of antigens available. This is one area in contact dermatitis where as-is testing to the crushed or powdered substance is not only possible but preferred and reliable—with the exception of a few acidic food sources (e.g., onion and garlic). It is important that immediate urticarial reactions not be overlooked. Further, in some cases, patch testing in the actual area of dermatitis is suggested if testing on the back is negative. The subject of contact urticaria has recently been summarized,[2] but there are a number of substances yet to be defined, and these are common causes of highly bothersome reactions in this industry.

In many of these food-, herb-, and spice-related sources of contact dermatitis, the site of involvement is not the hands but some other area where the individual commonly touches the body while performing the task at hand. Another consideration, often overlooked, is photo accentuation. A classic example is the blistering reactions from contact with celery. Photo testing is therefore to be considered if the distribution of the dermatitis suggests it and if hyperpigmentation is present. With proper instruction, patients can patch-test themselves if the history is not diagnostic. This is one situation in which I encourage this procedure and have my patch test technician available for any questions regarding procedures.

FLORISTS, NURSERYMEN, AND GARDENERS

The subject of botanical dermatology and contact dermatitis is even more voluminous than that covering the above occupational exposure. Further, the number of plant antigens available for patch testing is limited to a few well-known ones such as primin (see Appendix 1). Fortunately, patch testing to raw materials in this category is usually safe and rewarding—in fact, almost entertaining. There are certain well-known irritants, such as usnic acid, but if proper care is taken, testing is quite reliable. Once again, since the handling of most botanical materials involves getting the allergen embedded under the fingernails, severe allergic reactions will often occur at sites where the worker casually wipes off sweat or scratches, as is often seen in *Rhus* dermatitis.

As a rule, I do not suggest that patch testing be done routinely to poison ivy, oak, or sumac, as this may lead to sensitization to a commonly encountered allergen. For most other plants, one can simply take a small portion of the leaf, stem, and flower, crush these onto a 1- to 2-cm square of gauze, and apply the gauze to the back under occlusion for 48 hr. At the first sign of irritation or itching, the patch should be removed and examined by the patient; proper instruction is a must! Also, following removal of test patches, exposure to sunlight is suggested on a routine basis, since many of these reactions are either photo accentuated or are positive only with proper exposure to ultraviolet light. Such exposure can be done utilizing natural sunlight through window glass or even direct sunlight if care is taken to prevent burning. An excellent reference[13] is available which covers the broad plant kingdom, with appropriate photos and patch test suggestions. In testing nursery workers (Figure 6-1), where one is often dealing with more exotic and less well-known plant sources, a more exhaustive reference[14] is available.

Recently, a unique source of severe contact dermatitis with many disabling cases of hand dermatitis has resulted from exposure to *Alstroemeria* (Figures 6-2 and 6-3). The antigen involved, tuliposide A, has been identified

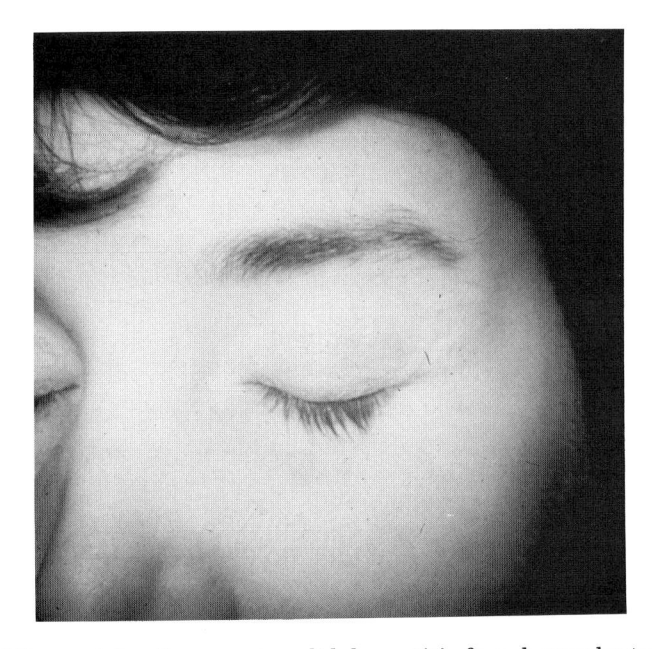

Figure 6-1. Recurrent eyelid dermatitis from houseplants.

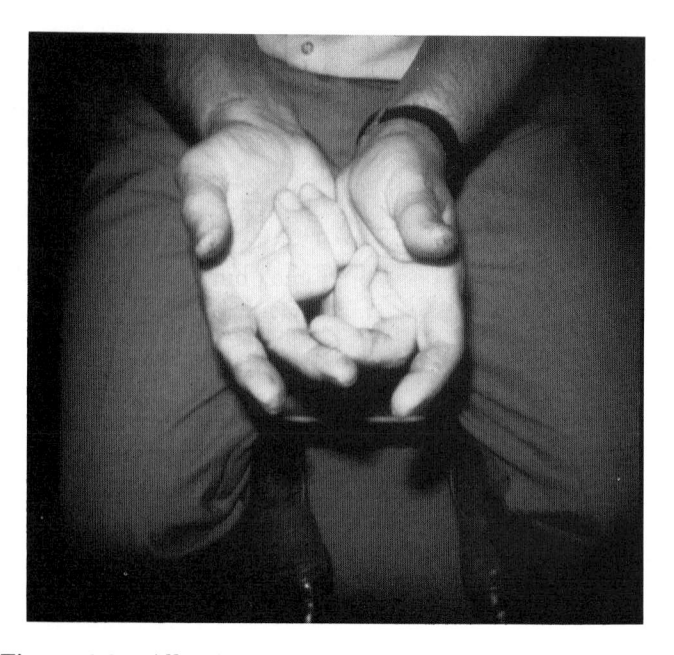

Figure 6-2. Allergic contact dermatitis due to *Alstroemeria*.

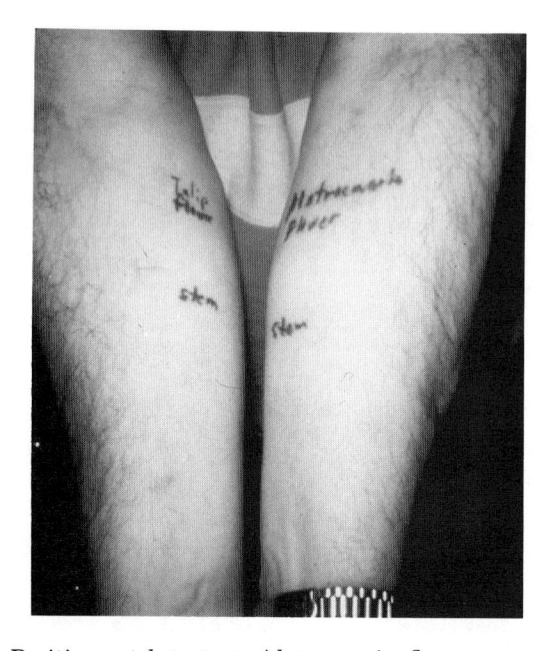

Figure 6-3. Positive patch tests to *Alstroemeria*, flower, stem, and tulip leaf.

and is available for testing. However, patch testing to this ornamental flower can be easily accomplished utilizing portions of the plant as outlined above. The evolution of knowledge regarding *Alstroemeria* and the inability of standard gloves to protect against this antigen provides a classic example of how information is often not disseminated to industry appropriately. Many, perhaps thousands, of florists suffer from this severe form of contact dermatitis due to lack of information regarding its allergenicity and protective measures. There is no ready answer to this dilemma, but certainly we should make a greater effort to communicate such information and prevent unnecessary exposure and sensitization to a potent allergen.

I would be remiss in not bringing up the subject of pesticides and fungicides, as well as other substances which are often applied to plants to preserve their natural beauty. It is my opinion that, except in certain intense exposure situations in agriculture-related settings, this is not a common cause of allergic contact dermatitis. This group of chemicals should be patch-tested carefully. I do not recommend as-is testing. The references previously given[1-3] provide excellent, up-to-date coverage of these materials.

CONSTRUCTION—IN THE BROAD SENSE

Most of the antigen exposure in construction workers, cabinet makers, bricklayers, and painters is fairly well established. In recent years, with the widespread incorporation of formaldehyde resins and fungicides to preserve wood products and improve paints and varnishes, a new element has been added to the spectrum of contact dermatitis in these occupations. The large variety of glues used in wood laminants and particle board has increased the exposure to these "additives." This is one area where patch testing to such things as sawdust is practical and expedient, but the basic irritating nature of cements, adhesives, and paints requires that testing be performed using the dried material. I usually encourage testing in this group of occupational contactants, and I would also include plastic laminants that are being increasingly utilized in this industry. A practical guideline is to patch-test to the pulverized, finished materials on a moist gauze pad and occlude for 48 hr.

A group requiring special consideration are those who perform decorative or ornamental woodworking (Figure 6-4). Some of these beautiful woods have been well outlined in references previously cited,[14] and careful history taking is key in suspecting them. When patch-testing to these materials, it is important to have the patient remove the test patch immediately if itching or irritation supervenes.

HAIRDRESSERS, COSMETICIANS, AND ESTHETICIANS

In keeping with modern grooming standards, a new source of contact allergy has emerged that relates to physical appearance, especially the skin, hair,

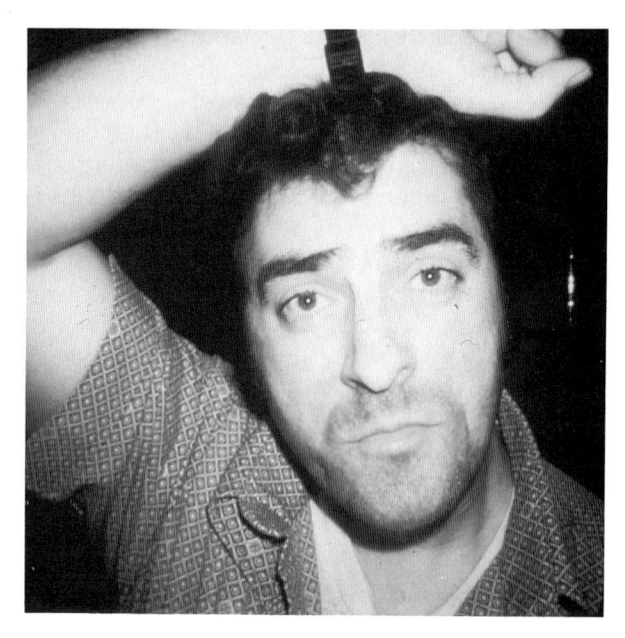

Figure 6-4. Airborne allergic contact dermatitis due to woods-walnut, juniper, and teak sanding dust.

and nails. Most reactions to hair care products have been well defined, but patch testing to the raw materials can be fraught with irritant reactions and both false negatives and false positives.[4] This is one area where I encourage dermatologists to utilize the standard trays which are available,[11,12] along with careful examination of the products brought in by the patient. In my experience, hairdressers rarely suspect the actual cause of their contact dermatitis. They, and often I, find it difficult to separate irritant from allergic dermatitis. Therefore, it is my premise that patch testing is always indicated if the dermatitis is chronic and/or disabling. If testing to standard trays is negative, it becomes imperative to scrutinize all contact sources. This is an area where a further history obtained by the dermatologist or the interested patch test technician can help.

The evolution of nail care products—artificial nails, silk wraps, and nail sculpturing—has resulted in the development of a number of interesting, strong sensitizers. This subject has recently been reviewed.[15] Most of these substances are available for routine patch testing, but patch testing to the product is possible if care is taken. I prefer to perform two tests: A small amount of the glue or polish is applied directly to the skin, allowed to dry thoroughly, and is then covered with a gauze pad. In addition, a small amount of the material is applied to a gauze pad, allowed to dry thoroughly, and applied to the skin for 48 hr. Patients are advised to remove either of the substances with acetone or nail polish remover if severe itching develops. Patch testing to the finished nail can also be performed, but many times the "cured" product will not produce a positive patch test in sensitized individuals.

It is important to keep in mind that consumers who become allergic to these nail care products and adhesives will often present with subungual pain or with recurrent candidiasis or bacterial infection of the periunguium. For this reason, contact dermatitis is not immediately suspected, especially since the patient does not have a significant history of itching. Further, since many of these rejections occur after months of use, other sources are often suspected. I believe that all hairdressers, cosmeticians, estheticians, and nail care specialists be patch-tested to standard, known contact allergens, as well as to all the materials they bring to the office.

TEXTILE WORKERS, KNITTERS, AND SEAMSTRESSES IN CONTACT WITH TEXTILE DYES AND FINISHES AND FORMALDEHYDE IN GENERAL

The subject of clothing dermatitis has recently been reviewed,[16] and it is becoming obvious that fabric finish and dye dermatitis is much more common than we have previously recognized. From an occupational standpoint, the dermatitis usually is related to the area where the finish or dye contacts the skin. Since the irritating nature of these chemicals is well known, protective gauntlett gloves often will spare the hands and the worker will present with dermatitis of the upper arms or neck, or even the abdomen and thighs where the wet material soaks through the clothing. The degree of dermatitis varies considerably from an irritant form—erythema, lichenification, and fissuring—to an acute eczematous dermatitis, often with secondary infection. Often workers and/or the attending physician fail to recognize the source; this leads to chronic dermatitis requiring prolonged therapy. In my experience, some of these *workers* experience itching, burning, and edema of the eyes and periorbital skin, as well as occasional episodes of sneezing or bronchial reactions related to the exposure. This is in contrast to *patients* with clothing/fabric dermatitis which involves the skin only, usually periaxillary, antecubital, and/or the lateral abdomen and waistband areas. In both workers and patients, no area of the skin that comes in contact with dyes or finishes should be overlooked; sources include upholstery, carpets, automobile seats, curtains, sewing materials, and any treated fabric.

As a rule, patch testing to actual fabric components is difficult, and often negative results are obtained. For fabric finishes, a piece of fabric can be soaked for 10 min in a small amount of water and the extract used for a 48-hr occlusive patch test. When a dye is suspect, it has been suggested that a small piece of fabric be exposed to acetone or ethyl alcohol as a solvent and the extract used for testing. However, most formaldehyde resins and disperse dyes are now available in standardized concentrations for routine patch testing, and I strongly suggest that they be used—both for textile workers and for patients suspected of having clothing/fabric dermatitis. The patch tests are usually strongly positive and leave little doubt as to the degree of allergy the worker/patient is demonstrating.

A final point regarding fabric finish contact dermatitis should be mentioned, namely, cross-reactivity between fabric finishes, formaldehyde, and formaldehyde-releasing preservatives that are found in many creams and lotions. It is generally agreed that using formaldehyde in the standard tray as a screening agent for fabric finish dermatitis is not to be encouraged. I agree with this, but it is my belief that all patients with textile-related dermatitis should be patch-tested to the complete group of formaldehyde-releasing agents, as well as to both 1% and 2% formaldehyde solutions, since combined allergy is not infrequent.[17] If such testing is negative but the association is still highly suspect, actual material from the worker's workplace should be obtained, along with the MSDS, and carefully evaluated before the worker is advised that the problem is not work related.

CLERICAL WORKERS, BANKERS, NEWSPAPER WRITERS, AND OTHERS IN CONTACT WITH PAPER

Of all the groups of industrial contacts I have mentioned, this one is the most difficult to evaluate. One reason, I believe, is that individuals in these occupations often either wash their hands frequently or use other cleaning solvents which promote the development of irritant and/or allergic contact dermatitis. Further, their work exposes them to well-known causes of allergic contact dermatitis in the form of rubber gloves or finger cots, paraphenylenediamine, cobalt in inks, many glues and adhesives, and, more recently, the wide variety of formaldehyde finishes and other agents that are being used to treat and preserve paper products. In my experience, testing workers to the materials they bring into the office has been uniformly disappointing. I perform these tests, since testing is safe and relatively easy, but I always test to the standard tray and check carefully regarding factors supporting an irritant, rather than an allergic, basis for the dermatitis.

SUMMARY

I hope that I have provided some guidelines on when patch testing may be done "as is" and when more sophisticated testing is indicated. It is becoming increasingly apparent that not all forms of contact dermatitis are eczematous and itchy. Fortunately, excellent journals and other references are available to guide us in evaluating these patients. We should not be frustrated or exasperated when these occupational patients appear with a bag full of items they feel are causing their dermatitis. Rather, we should devise an approach which will lead to successful identification of the cause of these cases of often severe, chronic contact dermatitis (Figures 6-5 and 6-6). With the identification of such antigens in industry, we also gain useful information regarding the source of dermatitis in the consumers who use them.

If I could choose from among the various allergens other than those in the standard tray, I would choose a cosmetic series, a textile dyes and finishes series, and an acrylate and glue series—all of which are available from sources previously cited[11,12] (see Appendix 1). Obviously, the dermatologist who is

SUMMARY 79

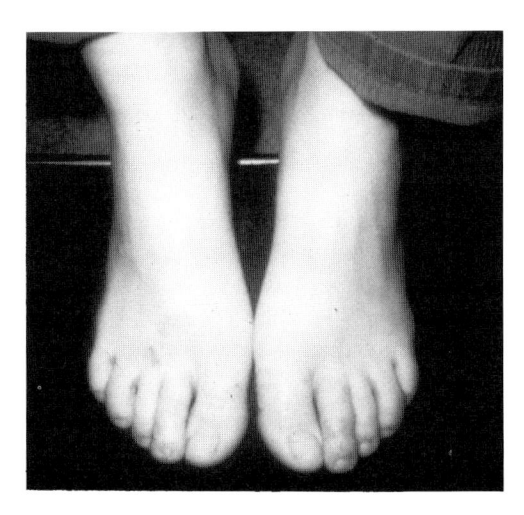

Figure 6-5. Allergic contact dermatitis due to athletic shoes.

dealing with a large population in a specific industry may wish to acquire one of the other series or, better yet, to prepare a personal series based on specific antigen exposure. Lastly, I should mention that contact dermatitis from corticosteroids is becoming increasingly apparent and has recently been reviewed.[18] It is obvious that almost all patients, whether treated by a dermatologist or a general practitioner, have probably used one or more topical steroids. As this source becomes further studied as a cause of allergic contact dermatitis, the necessary antigens which should be incorporated into standard or other trays will become apparent. For now, there is no single steroid antigen to which patients should be tested, and I suggest that patch testing be performed to all standardized antigens currently available.

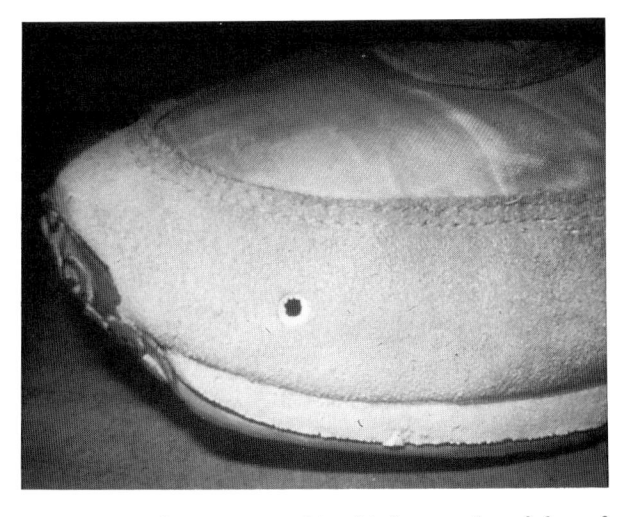

Figure 6-6. 6 or 8 mm punches suggested to obtain samples of shoes for patch testing.

REFERENCES

1. Adams RM: *Occupational Skin Disease.* Philadelphia, Grune & Stratton, 1990.
2. Maibach HI (ed): *Occupation and Industrial Dermatology.* Chicago, Year Book Medical, 1987.
3. Fossereau J, Benezra C, Maibach HI: *Occupational Contact Dermatitis: Clinical and Chemical Aspects.* Copenhagen, Munksgaard, 1982.
4. Fisher AA: *Contact Dermatitis,* ed 3. Philadelphia, Lea & Febiger, 1986.
5. Cronin E: *Contact Dermatitis.* New York, Churchill, Livingstone, 1980.
6. Fregert S: *Manual of Contact Dermatitis,* ed 2. Copenhagen, Munksgaard, 1981.
7. deGrooth AC: *Patch Testing. Test Concentrations and Vehicles for 2800 Allergens.* New York, Oxford University Press, 1986.
8. Jackson EM, Goldner R: *Irritant Contact Dermatitis.* New York, Marcel Decker, 1990.
9. Hamahn CP: Natural latex rubber protein sensitivity in review. *Am J Contact Dermatitis* 4:4–21, 1993.
10. Taylor JA, Melton A, Hamahn CP: Selected highlights of the International Latex Conference: Sensitivity to latex in medical devices, Baltimore, MD, November 5–7, *Am J Contact Dermatitis* 4:101–105, 1993.
11. Dormer Laboratories, Inc, 6600 Trans Canada Highway, Suite 750, Pointe Claire, Canada, Quebec H9R 454; telephone: (514) 451-0773.
12. Omniderm, Inc, 8400 Dornley Road, Montreal, Quebec, Canada, H4T 1M4; telephone: (514) 340-1114.
13. Benezra C, Ducombs G, Sell Y: *Plant Contact Dermatitis.* St Louis, CV Mosby, 1985.
14. Mitchell JC, Rook A: *Botanical Dermatology.* Vancouver, British Columbia, Canada, Greengrass, 1979.
15. Rosenweig R, Scher RK: Nail cosmetics: Adverse reactions. *Am J Contact Dermatitis* 4:71–77, 1993.
16. Sheretz EF: Clothing dermatitis: Practical aspects for the clinician. *Am J Contact Dermatitis* 3:56–64, 1992.
17. Daily A: Cross reactivity in patients with formaldehyde resin clothing dermatitis, presentation, Annual Meeting of American Contact Dermatitis Society, Washington, DC, Dec. 3, 1993.
18. Lauerma-Antti I: Contact hypersensitivity to glucocorticosteroids. *Am J Contact Dermatitis* 3:112–132, 1992.

7

Contact Urticaria

Chuchai Tanglertsampan
Howard I. Maibach

INTRODUCTION

The contact urticaria syndrome was defined as a biologic entity in 1975.[1] Subsequently, especially in the last decade, it has attracted increasing interest in clinical medicine and biology. Numerous cases have been published and provide new information on the etiologies and the clinical and pathophysiologic features of the syndrome. Extensive reviews have been published by Odom and Maibach, von Krogh and Maibach, and Lahti and Maibach.[2-4] This review covers the basic information for practicing dermatologists and updates the recent literature on contact urticaria. Latex protein contact urticaria is discussed separately.

DEFINITION

Immediate contact reactions of the skin are a heterogeneous group of inflammatory reactions that appear after contact with the eliciting substance. They include not only wheal and flare reactions, but also transient erythematous and eczematous reactions.

There has been much confusion in using terms such as *contact urticaria, immediate contact reactions, atopic contact dermatitis,* and *protein contact dermatitis* (Table 7-1). *Immediate contact reaction* includes both urticarial and other reactions, whereas *protein contact dermatitis* refers to allergic or nonallergic eczematous dermatitis caused by proteins or proteinaceous materials.

TABLE 7-1 Terminology of Immediate Contact Reactions

Term	Remarks
Immediate contact reaction	Includes urticarial, eczematous, and other immediate reactions
Contact urticaria	Allergic and nonallergic contact urticaria reactions
Protein contact dermatitis	Allergic or nonallergic eczematous reactions caused by proteins or proteinaceous material
Atopic contact dermatitis	Immediate urticarial or eczematous, IgE-mediated immediate contact reaction
Contact urticaria syndrome	Includes both local and systemic immediate reactions precipitated by contact urticaria agents (immunologic and nonimmunologic types)

Contact urticaria syndrome comprises both local and systemic immediate reactions precipitated by contact urticarial agents.

The mechanisms underlying contact reactions are divided into two main types, namely, immunological (IgE-mediated) and nonimmunological contact reactions.[5] However, there are also substances that cause immediate contact reactions whose mechanism may not be known (e.g., ammonium persulfate).

SYMPTOMS

Immediate contact reactions appear on normal or eczematous skin within minutes to hours after agents capable of producing these types of reactions come in contact with the skin. They disappear within 24 hr, usually within a few hours. The symptoms can be classified according to morphology and severity: itching, tingling, or burning accompanied by erythema are the weakest type of immediate contact reaction, and are often produced by cosmetics, fruits, and vegetables.[6] Local wheal-and-flare is the prototypical reaction of contact urticaria. Generalized urticaria after local contact is rare but can occur with strong urticant allergens. Tiny vesicles frequently appear on the fingers in protein contact dermatitis. Apart from the skin, effects may appear in other organs in cases of very strong hypersensitivity. In some cases, immediate contact reactions can be demonstrated only on slightly or previously affected skin and can be part of the mechanism responsible for maintenance of chronic eczemas.[7–9]

DIAGNOSTIC TESTS

The diagnosis of immediate contact reactions is based on a full medical history and on skin tests with suspected substances. If there is a risk of anaphylaxis a radioallergosorbent test (RAST) may be performed before skin testing. Suggested test procedures for evaluation of immediate responses are provided in

TABLE 7-2 Suggested Test Procedures for Evaluation of Immediate Responses

Type of Test	Need for Controls
1. Epidermal	

A. Open application (noninvasive)
    Nonaffected (normal) skin
    ↓ negative / ↓ positive*
    Slightly affected (previously affected) skin
    ↓ negative / ↓ positive*
	Minimal

B. Occlusive application (patch or chamber)
    Nonaffected (normal) skin
    ↓ negative / ↓ positive*
    Slightly affected (previously affected) skin
    ↓ negative / ↓ positive*
	Increased

2. Dermal: Invasive (prick, scratch, or intradermal injection)	Strong, especially with scratch or intradermal testing

*If positive reactions are obtained, discontinue further evaluation.

Table 7-2. It is emphasized that very low concentrations of allergens should be used for testing in immunological contact urticaria when the history indicates that extracutaneous organs are involved. Resuscitation facilities should be immediately available.

CAUSES

Selected causes of occupational contact urticaria are presented in Table 7-3.[10] Recently reported causes of contact urticaria are tabulated in Table 7-4.

TABLE 7-3 Selected Causes of Occupational Contact Urticaria

Agent	Nonimmunologic	Immunologic
Animals	Caterpillars Jellyfish, corals Moths	Animal products (e.g., placenta, saliva) Cockroaches, wool
Foods	Cayenne pepper Fish Mustard Thyme	Cheese, egg, milk Kiwi, mango, banana Maize, beans, peanut butter Sesame foods, sunflower seeds Beef, chicken, lamb, liver, turkey Seafood (e.g., fish, prawns, shrimp)
Fragrances and flavorings	Balsam of Peru Cassia (cinnamon oil) Cinnamic acid Cinnamic aldehyde	Balsam of Peru Menthol Vanillin

Medications	Alcohols
	Benzocaine
	Camphor
	Capsaicin
	Dimethyl sulfoxide
	Friar's balsam
	Nicotinic acid esters
	Tar extracts
	Tincture of benzoin
		Antibiotics
		  Ampicillin
		  Bacitracin
		  Cephalosporins
		  Gentamycin
		  Iodochlorhyroxyquine
		  Neomycin
		  Penicillin
		  Rifampin
		  Streptomycin
		  Virginiamycin
		Benzocaine
		Phenothiazines
		  Chlorpromazine
		  Levomepromazine
		  Promethazine

Plants	Nettles
	Seaweed
		Plant products
		  Colophony
		  Cornstarch
		  Henna
		  Latex rubber
		  Lime
		  Teak
		  Tulip

Preservatives and disinfectants	Benzoic acid Chlorocresol Formaldehyde Sodium benzoate Sorbic acid	Benzoic acid Benzyl alcohol Castor bean Chlorhexidine Chlorocresol Formaldehyde Gentian violet Sodium hypochlorite
Miscellaneous	Ammonium persulfate Benzophenone Histamine Sulfur Turpentine	Alcohols Carbonless copying paper Epoxy resin Formaldehyde resin Nickel Paraphenylenediamine Seminal fluid

TABLE 7-4 Recently Reported Causes of Contact Urticaria

Category	Substance Name	No. of Cases	History Derm.	History Extraderm.	Test Immediate	Test Delay	Control	Classification
Chemical industry	Acrylic acid (2-propenic a.)	1	GU		Open		6	ND
Dyes	Reactive dyes	3	LU?	Resp	Scratch/Scratch chamber/Prick		10	ICU
Medication	Diphenycyclopropenone	4	GU		Open?		No	ND
	Nicotine base/sulfate	8	LU?		Open		No	ND
Metal	Mercuric fluorescein comp.	2	GU	AR?	Prick		10	ICU?
Plant	Bougainvillaea	1	LU		Scratch chamber		10	ND
	Phaseolus multiflorus (Runner bean)	1	LU		Prick		10	ND
	Triplochiton scleroxylon	8			Prick		Yes**	ICU
	Eruca sativa	1	LU		Prick		5	ICU
	Semecarpus anaacardium	1	LU		Open		10	ND
Textiles Tinofix S®	Formaldehyde Dicyandiamide Amm. Chloride Ethylenediamine etc.*	1	LU	AR	Open		3	ND
Miscellaneous	Hypochlorite	1	GU?	Resp.	Open		No	ICU
	1,1,1-Trichloroethan	1	LU		Closed patch		6	ND

LU = localized urticaria; GU = generalized urticaria; AR = anaphylactoid reaction; Resp = respiratory system; ICU = immunologic contact urticaria; ND = not determined; * = no specific allergens determined; ** = numbers of controls are not provided.

85

Most initial clinical judgments hypothesized in the report by Maibach and Johnson[1] have been subsequently largely confirmed. It is crucial for the dermatologist to recognize immediate contact reactions and to be able to perform appropriate immediate type skin tests. In clinical practice, patients report immediate contact reactions after applying cosmetics or therapeutic agents and after handling food products. There are many unsolved issues in understanding this type of reaction and in developing less urticarsogenic products. Important technical changes in mechanistic evaluation have been the increasing utilization of the RAST test and decreasing use of passive transfer testing in humans, the latter because of concern regarding inadvertent transfer of infectious diseases.

Controls

It is our judgment that few controls are requisite with open testing; hence our enthusiasm for the practical aspects of its utilization. However, with open testing, it is sometimes essential to apply the putative responsible agent to the involved anatomical sites or to slightly damaged skin rather than to the forearm.[9,11] Any response to a chemical that is producing an immediate flare and/or wheal and flare is by definition a contact urticaria; however, a positive open test does not identify the mechanism, for example, nonimmunologic contact urticaria (NICU) versus immunologic contact urticaria (ICU). Separation of these mechanisms requires further evaluation according to the algorithm given in Table 7-5.

The issue of controls in prick and scratch tests requires emphasis. In the recent literature,[12-14] 10 controls have sometimes been provided. More controls should be used, especially with scratch testing, as many materials produce positive reactions in a nonimmunologic manner. Normal saline or other appropriate diluents may be used for prick or scratch testing controls. It is crucial to begin with very diluted allergen concentrations and use serial dilutions, if required, for skin testing to minimize allergen exposure when extracutaneous manifestations are expected. The precautions for the treatment of anaphylaxis must be maintained.

TABLE 7-5   ICU vs. NICU

Characteristics	ICU	NICU
1. PK test*	Positive	Not relevant
2. RAST test	Positive	Negative
3. Occurrence at first exposure	No	Yes
4. Open test in controls	Negative	Positive in many to most cases

*Prausnitz-Kustner test.

CONTACT URTICARIA FROM LATEX PROTEIN

Natural rubber latex protein sensitivity has recently been reviewed by Hamann.[15] Nutter first reported an urticarial reaction to natural rubber latex in 1979.[16] It is a crucial and frequent problem, especially in health care workers. Turjanmaa reported natural rubber latex protein prevalence at a teaching hospital in Finland in which 7.4% of surgeons and 5.6% of surgical nurses had a positive scratch chamber test.[17] There is a significantly increased prevalence among females, atopic patients (particularly those with chronic hand eczema), spina bifida patients, patients who have had multiple surgeries or instrumentation of the genitourinary tract during infancy, and health care providers exposed frequently to natural rubber latex. Natural latex is an intracellular milky fluid produced by lacticifier cells of the tropical rubber tree *Hevea brasiliensis*. Antigens in the regions of 14 kd and 30 kd seem to be most reproducible.[15] For a discussion of symptoms and diagnostic testing, please see the previous sections.

Management

Persons with a positive IgE-specific RAST, prick, or use test are treated with complete natural rubber latex avoidance. Although hypoallergic natural rubber latex gloves, powder-free natural rubber latex gloves, dry rubber latex gloves, or synthetic polymer-lined natural rubber latex gloves may be appropriate recommendations for patients with delayed hypersensitivity reactions, these gloves may still contain sufficient natural rubber latex protein to elicit an anaphylactic reaction.[18,19] Vinyl, choloropene, nitrile, or Tactyl (Smart Practice, Phoenix, Arizona, USA) alternatives should be substituted for individuals with diagnosed natural rubber latex protein hypersensitivity. The term *hypoallergenic*, used in conjunction with latex gloves, initially referred only to natural rubber latex gloves with a reduced type IV antigen content. When health care providers are severely sensitized, they should avoid working in an environment with colleagues who wear powdered natural rubber latex gloves because of the increased risk of anaphylaxis from cornstarch airborne natural rubber latex protein. Probably just as important as avoiding natural rubber latex are measures to prevent sensitization where the incidence appears greatest. Atopic health care workers with chronic eczema should avoid natural rubber latex when possible. Similarly, children with spina bifida who are undergoing multiple surgeries and multiple catheterizations during their first years of life should minimize the risk of sensitization with natural rubber latex avoidance.

REFERENCES

1. Maibach HI, and Johnson HL. Contact urticaria syndrome: Contact urticaria to diethytoluamide (immediate type hypersensitivity). *Arch Dermatol* 111:726, 1975.

2. Odom RB, and Maibach HI. Contact urticaria: A different contact dermatitis, in Marzulli FN, Maibach HI (eds), *Dermatotoxicology and Pharmacology,* Cutis, 1976, pp 672–676.
3. von Krogh G, and Maibach HI. The contact urticaria syndrome—an update review. *J Am Acad Dermatol* 5:328, 1981.
4. Lahti A, Maibach HI. Immediate contact reactions: Contact urticaria and contact urticaria syndrome, in Marzulli FN, Maibach HI (eds), *Dermatotoxicology.* Hemisphere, 1991, pp 473–495.
5. Lahti A, Maibach HI. Immediate contact reactions: Contact urticaria syndrome. *Semin Dermatol* 6:313, 1987.
6. Emmons WW, Marks JG. Immediate and delayed reactions to cosmetic ingredients. *Contact Dermatitis* 13:258, 1985.
7. Hannuksela M. Atopic contact dermatitis. *Contact Dermatitis* 6(1)30, 1980.
8. Veien NK, Hattel T, Justesen O, et al. Dietary restrictions in the treatment of adult patients with eczema. *Contact Dermatitis* 17:223, 1987.
9. Maibach HI. Immediate hypersensitivity in hand dermatitis: Role of food contact dermatitis. *Arch Dermatol* 112:1289, 1976.
10. Hogan DJ, Tanglertsampan C. The less common occupational dermatoses. *State of the Art Review: Occupational Medicine* 7:385, 1992.
11. Maibach HI. Regional variation in elicitation of contact urticaria syndrome (immediate hypersensitivity syndrome): Shrimp. *Contact Dermatitis* 15:100, 1986.
12. Estlander T. Allergic dermatoses and respiratory diseases from reactive dyes. *Contact Dermatitis* 18:290, 1988.
13. Sanz B, Munoz FT, Serrano LC, et al. Hypersensitivity to mercuric fluorescein compounds. *Allergol Immnopathol* 17:219, 1989.
14. Shankar DSK. Contact urticaria induced by *Semecarpus anacardium. Contact Dermatitis* 26:200, 1992.
15. Hamann CP. Natural rubber latex protein sensitivity in review. *Am J Contact Dermatitis* 4:4, 1993.
16. Nutter AF. Contact urticaria to rubber. *Br J Dermatol* 101:597, 1979.
17. Turjanmaa K. Incidence of immediate allergy to latex gloves in hospital personnel. *Contact Dermatitis* 17:270, 1987.
18. Frosch PJ, Wahl R, Bahmer FA, et al. Contact urticaria to rubber gloves is IgE-mediated. *Contact Dermatitis* 14:241, 1986.
19. Warpinski JR, Folgret J, Cohen M, et al. Allergic reaction to latex. An unsuspected risk factor for anaphylaxis. *Allergy Pract* 12:95, 1991.

8

Other Occupational Dermatoses: Acne, Pigmentary Disorders, Skin Cancer, Infection, Reactions to Temperature and Humidity, Scleroderma, and Nail Changes

Tamra A. Ruxin and James S. Taylor

INTRODUCTION

Contact dermatitis accounts for the vast majority of occupational skin disorders. However, the nondermatitic occupational dermatoses are also important. Those included in this chapter are acne, pigmentary disorders, skin cancer, infections, reactions to temperature and humidity, scleroderma, and nail disorders. Many occur infrequently; examples include chloracne and scleroderma due to workplace exposures. Others are more common; examples include miliaria and postinflammatory hyperpigmentation. For coverage of other uncommon nondermatitic occupational disorders, the reader is referred to other sources.[1,2]

ACNE

Occupational acne results from contact with petroleum and its derivatives, coal tar products, and certain halogenated aromatic hydrocarbons. The eruption may be mild and localized or extensive, involving most follicular orifices. It may be aggravated by heat, friction, excessive scrubbing, cosmetics, pomade, and topical corticosteroids.[3]

Petroleum-Induced Acne

Petroleum-induced acne is most commonly seen in mechanics exposed to grease and lubricating oils, as well as in workers exposed to cutting oils in the machine tool trades, where the insoluble (straight) oils and semisynthetic metal working fluids are the most frequent causes. Comedones and inflammatory folliculitis of the dorsa of the hands and extensor surfaces of the forearms are typical of oil acne; however, covered areas of the body, especially the thighs, lower abdomen, and buttocks, may be affected by contact with oil-saturated clothing.[3]

Coal Tar–Induced Acne

Coal tar oil-, creosote-, and pitch-induced acne is most commonly seen in coal tar plant workers, roofers, road maintenance workers, and construction workers. Coal tar acne typically presents with comedones, but phototoxic reactions of the skin and eye (keratoconjunctivitis) may complicate the picture.[3] Pitch kerotoses and acanthomas may appear subsequently.

Environmental Halogen Acne (Chloracne)

Environmental halogen acne, frequently called *chloracne,* is caused by halogenated aromatic chemicals having a specific molecular shape.[4-16] Most cases have been due to trace contaminants of herbicides, herbicide intermediates, polychlorinated biphenyls (PCBs), and flame retardants. Most clinical and experimental studies have identified these contaminants as 2,3,7,8-tetrachlorodibenzo-para-dioxin (TCDD), polyhalogenated dibenzofurans, polyhalogenated biphenyls, azoxybenzenes, azobenzenes, and congeners. Polyhalogenated naphthalenes, potent acnegens once used in the electronics industry as insulating waxes, may also occur as contaminants of polychlorobiphenyls and polybromobiphenyls.[5] TCDD is the best-studied and most potent acnegenic compound and is formed during the synthesis of the herbicide intermediate 2,4,5-trichlorphenol. Symptoms of acute exposure to TCDD include nausea, vomiting, headache, and respiratory and eye irritation. Skin irritation probably results from sodium trichlorophenate burns of exposed skin areas rather than from TCDD exposure.[6] Chronic sequelae of TCDD exposure include chloracne, porphyria cutanea tarda, hyperpigmentation and hypertrichosis without porphyria, psychiatric disturbances, and neuromuscular, central nervous system, liver, kidney, and pancreatic disease.[3] Exposure may occur through accidental industrial exposure of workers, uncontrolled release into the atmosphere as a result of an industrial accident, and spraying of contaminated material into the environment.[4] Combustion of industrial waste and fires, as well as explosions of PCB-containing electrical transformers, have produced TCDD and tetrachlorodibenzofurans.[7,8]

Chloracne typically presents with comedones as the basic and only lesions in mild cases. As evidence of toxicity increases, characteristic straw-colored cysts appear. Inflammatory pustules and abscesses may also occur. The distribution commonly includes the malar crescent, postauricular area, cheeks, forehead, and neck in order of frequency. When extensive, chloracne involves the shoulders, chest, back, penis, scrotum, buttocks, abdomen, and axilla. The nose is frequently spared.[7] Axillary lesions have been seen in patients in whom ingestion or inhalation was known to be a major route of absorption, as in the nonoccupational cases of PCB ingestion in Japan and Taiwan or TCDD environmental exposure in Seveso, Italy.[8] PCBs may be passed transplacentally from mother to fetus, with nail dystrophy and nail bed pigmentation as the main cutaneous evidence of PCB exposure.[9]

Accompanying or preceding cutaneous signs may point to certain chemical causes, including hyperpigmentation with TCDD and PCB exposure, acute burns, facial edema with 2,4,5-trichlorophenol accidents, actinic elastosis with TCDD exposure, and Meibomian gland cysts with PCB exposure.[4,5,7,8] Although porphyria may be induced in laboratory animals by certain chloracnegenic chemicals, it has been infrequently identified in exposed humans. Hepatic porphyria from TCDD has been described at least twice in humans, but exposure was mixed, with multiple possible causative agents.[4,5] Chemical porphyria may be more common than clinical porphyria, but its use as an indicator of disease is questionable.[4]

Histologically, in chloracne, sebaceous glands are replaced by keratin cysts, which always have an attachment to the epidermis. Crow believes that this "rapid and total transformation of sebaceous glands into squamous cysts is pathognomonic to poisoning with chloracnegens and is of the greatest diagnostic value."[8] However, while this may be true when one examines a series of cases, differentiation from acne vulgaris may be difficult or impossible in mild, isolated cases.[5] Clinical differentiation from solar comedones may also be difficult.[2,5] Eccrine sweat duct horny metaplasia in the Seveso children exposed to TCDD suggests that sweat glands are one route of chloracnegen elimination.[10]

Chloracne tends to be refractory to treatment, and the lesions may continue to appear even after all exposure to the inciting chemical has ceased, resulting from chemical release from fat or hepatic stores.[5] Chloracne has been shown to be clinically reversible, as noted on a follow-up study of patients exposed to TCDD after an accidental spill in Seveso.[11] Oral antibiotics, acne surgery, topical tretinoin, and, more recently, oral 13-cis-retinoic acid are the main therapeutic options in treating chloracne. Zugerman[4] cites Tucker as stating that early institution of retinoid therapy may prevent cyst formation.

While chloracne is the hallmark of dioxin exposure, Silbergeld argues that "its absence is not proof that no toxicologically significant exposure has taken place."[12] Not all workers exposed to TCDD developed chloracne.[12,13] A recent study comparing blood levels of TCDD in workers with and without chloracne considered chloracne to be a reliable indicator of heavy dioxin exposure in a cohort of herbicide production workers.[14] Recent studies have addressed issues of occupational exposure limits[15] and dose–response models for TCDD.[16]

PIGMENTARY DISORDERS

Hyperpigmentation

Occupationally induced hyperpigmentation, the most common work-related pigment change,[17] may result from a postinflammatory event, chemical photosensitivity, nonphotosensitive chemical exposure, physical agents, or trauma. Chemical photosensitizers include tar, pitch, dyes, drugs, antimicrobial agents, and phototoxic oils and fragrances.[3] Phototoxic plants include parsnip, celery, lime, fig, mustard, and buckwheat.

Chemicals such as arsenic and certain acnegenic halogenated, aromatic hydrocarbons may lead to hyperpigmentation without photosensitization. Occupational arsenic exposure may be found in the following workers: agricultural, rodenticide, pesticide, copper and lead smelter, utility, semiconductor, printing ink, and leather workers and painters.[18,19] Arsenic exposure in the workplace may also occur through respiratory absorption while smoking or through ingestion while eating on the job. Skin absorption is a much less prevalent portal of entry for arsenic, but systemic toxic effects, as well as local skin inflammation, irritation, vesiculation, and folliculitis, have been reported following accidental spills of arsenic acid or arsenic trichloride.[20] Hyperpigmentation is the most frequently observed clinical response to chronic arsenic poisoning. Lesions are dark brown macules or patches present at sites of normally increased pigmentation such as the axilla, groin, or areola.[18] Various degrees of hypopigmentation have also been described.[21] Arsenical hyperpigmentation results from melanin deposition, not from arsenic deposition in the skin.[22]

The mechanism of hyperpigmentation from the acnegenic halogenated, aromatic hydrocarbons is unclear and is probably not a postinflammatory event. It is usually confined to the face, although it may become generalized in severe poisoning.[7] Hyperpigmentation has been reported from TCDD and PCB exposures. Japanese and Tawainese cases of PCB poisoning from ingestion of contaminated rice-based cooking oil were also associated with nail and mucosal (lips, gingiva, buccal, and conjunctival) pigmentation. Similar pigmentation affecting the nails and conjunctiva has been found in industrial PCB poisoning, but only in 2–3% of cases.[5,7,8]

Physical agents causing hyperpigmentation include ultraviolet light, as well as thermal and ionizing radiation. The affected areas typically involve those directly exposed to these agents. A number of industrial chemicals may stain the skin. These stains serve as markers of cutaneous exposure when symptoms of systemic toxicity are present in the absence of an obvious history of exposure. Orange stains have been produced by nitric acid, trinitrotoluene, dinitrophenol, and metaphenylenediamine.[23] Discoloration can be produced by a number of other chemicals.[21]

Hypopigmentation

Occupational pigment loss may result from chemical, thermal, or ultraviolet radiation burns or from postinflammatory changes, both of which involve the destruction of pigment-forming cells in the affected area. Occupational leukoderma may also result from cutaneous exposure to a variety of phenolic or catecholic derivatives which resemble tyrosine, a precursor of melanin synthesis. According to Mathias, at low doses these substances simply inhibit melanin synthesis, but at higher doses they may be cytotoxic to melanocytes.[23] Chemical leukoderma may appear identical to vitiligo, with confetti-like small, round to oval grouped macules and with a similar anatomic distribution and histologic findings. Chemical leukoderma usually follows direct contact, but inhalation or ingestion may also be operative. Exposure occurs during a 2-week to 6-month period, with cases commonly clustered in a factory.[24] Chemical irritation or sensitization is not a prerequisite for depigmentation. Spontaneous pigment return has been reported in some cases.[1] In our limited experience, psoralen plus ultraviolet A (PUVA) works well if it is used soon after the diagnosis of leukoderma is made and if the chemical insult is mild.

Chemical leukoderma was first reported in 1939 from monobenzylether of hydroquinone (MBEH), present as an antioxidant in industrial gloves. MBEH is now rarely used in industry. Related chemicals producing pigment loss include hydroquinone, monomethyl ether of hydroquinone (*p*-methoxyphenol or *p*-hydroxyanisole), and monoethylether of hydroquinone (*p*-ethoxyphenol). Hydroquinone rarely produces complete depigmentation, does not produce pigment loss at distant sites, as does MBEH, and is a weaker allergen than MBEH.[25] Other causes of chemical leukoderma include the alkylphenols, used industrially as antioxidants or rust inhibitors, and in deodorants, disinfectants, germicides, insecticides, lubricating and motor oils, paints, petroleum products, photographic chemicals, plastics and resins, printing inks, and synthetic rubber.[17] A simple review of ingredients in chemical formulations may be inadequate to detect the presence of chemicals inducing leukoderma, as the synthesis of by-products may form phenolic or catecholic depigmenting derivatives. In this situation, gas chromatographic analysis is required.[26]

SKIN CANCER

Occupationally linked skin cancers include squamous cell carcinoma, basal cell carcinoma, and possibly malignant melanoma. Chacteristically, tumors appear only after long-term exposure (at least 10 to 25 years) in a related occupation and may occur after a worker leaves the causal occupation. In some cases, the incubation period is shorter. Occupationally induced skin cancers tend to occur at a younger age than nonoccupationally induced cancers and the lesions are more likely to be multiple, with well-defined precancerous lesions typically preceding such skin cancers.[27] The etiology of such cancers includes exposure to polycyclic aromatic hydrocarbons, inorganic arsenic, ultraviolet light, and ionizing radiation. Trauma and burns, common occurrences in some occupations, have also been implicated in the development of skin cancers.[1] Work-related chemical exposure should be suspected when a squamous or basal cell carcinoma arises on skin that is not chronically exposed to sunlight.[23]

Polycyclic Hydrocarbons

The first occupationally related skin cancer was noted in 1775 by Percival Pott, an English surgeon, who drew attention to scrotal cancer in adolescent chimney sweeps; scrotal cancer is now known to be associated with the high content of 3,4-benzpyrene in soot.[27] Twenty years after Dr. Pott implicated soot, tar was suspected as a cause of lip cancer,[28] and by 1876, shale oil was also recognized as a carcinogenic agent.[27]

The most common chemical causes of occupational skin cancer are polycyclic hydrocarbons, which include 3,4-benzpyrene, dibenzanthracene, 3-methylcholanthrene, and 7,12-dimethylbenzanthracene. These chemicals are found in soot, pitch, coal tar, and creosote, as well as in shale, mineral, petroleum, and cutting oils.[27] Workers at risk include chimney sweeps, tar distillers, coal gas and briquette manufacturers, roofers, road builders, carbon black makers, timber picklers, shoemakers, cotton mule spinners, mineral oil users, machinists, and shale oil, refinery, paraffin, and rubber workers.[18] The Cancer Surveillance Program of the New York State Department of Health considers skin cancer of the scrotum to be a sentinel health event which is necessarily occupationally related.[29]

Besides the scrotum, skin cancer may develop on the face, ears, legs, and exposed forearms and hands. A precancerous, warty growth usually precedes the development of these nonmelanoma skin cancers.[27,30] There are at present no set standards for polyaromatic hydrocarbon exposure, so that good cutaneous hygiene minimizing skin contact, along with worker education, is most important.[18]

Inorganic Arsenic

Inorganic arsenic is another well-documented agent associated with occupationally induced skin cancer. As discussed in the section on hyperpigmentation, there are many industries where arsenic poisoning is a potential risk. Arsenic is unique in that skin tumors may be produced by ingestion, injection, or inhalation, not requiring skin contact, as do most other cutaneous carcinogens.[18] Arsenic has also been implicated in cancers of the bladder, kidney, lung, and liver.[31]

Arsenical keratoses typically appear on the palms and soles and may become generalized, potentially progressing to squamous cell or basal cell carcinoma.[3] Arsenic-induced skin cancers are often multiple and occur in non-sun-exposed areas. They do not differ histologically from nonarsenic-related tumors, but they do appear to be more clinically aggressive.[18] The arsenic exposure standard presently in effect limits the allowed exposure to 0.5 mg/m^3 in air for an 8-hr time-weighted average. This is higher than the proposed permissible exposure limit proposed by the Occupational Health and Safety Administration (OSHA) and does not address exposure through ingestion in workers eating and smoking in the work area.[18]

Ultraviolet Light

The most common cause of precancers and cancers of the skin is excess ultraviolet light exposure. Workers with outdoor occupations such as farmers, construction workers, ranchers, fishcatchers, sailors, highway patrol officers, and utility workers may be at increased risk for precancerous actinic keratoses potentially progressing to squamous cell carcinomas. Other findings in highly sun-exposed workers include hyperpigmentation, telangiectasias, and wrinkled skin.[1] Predisposing risk factors in the development of ultraviolet light–induced cancer include fair skin, increased susceptibility to sunburn, and Northern European ancestry.[23] Prevention of skin cancer in Australian outdoor workers was attempted through educational materials and audiovisual programs, and led to an improvement in overall protection from sunlight in these workers.[32] The educational program included posters and a video about a young man dying of melanoma, as well as a folder of material for each worker.

Ionizing Radiation

Ionizing radiation was associated with skin cancer shortly after Roentgen discovered X-rays in 1895.[27] Workers at risk are those with increased exposure to ionizing radiation and include technicians, physicians, dentists, and occupations involved with radiation-cured plastics, nuclear power plants, and sterilization of medical materials.[27] Direct exposure may induce squamous or basal cell carcinomas. The best protection is gained by minimizing exposure, monitoring radiation doses with ring or pin badges, and remaining aware of one's own radiation exposure level.[33]

Malignant Melanoma

Malignant melanoma has been reported to be occupationally related in some cases. Excessive exposure to sunlight in outdoor occupations has been linked to malignant melanomas of the head, face, neck, and all sun-exposed areas.[34,35] The incidence of malignant melanoma has been noted to be higher in the printing industry, specifically in typographers and workers in the newspaper printing industry.[36] Polycyclic hydrocarbons have also been implicated in excessive deaths from malignant melanoma.[18] Workers at the Lawrence Livermore National Laboratory were noted to have a threefold increase in the incidence of cutaneous malignant melanoma since 1972; however, an occupational cause has not yet been identified. The increased diagnosis of early malignant melanomas is now possible.[37,38]

INFECTIONS

The list of occupationally acquired infections is virtually limitless, as exposure to certain viral, bacterial, fungal, and parasitic agents is more likely in a wide variety of work. Since biological pathogens abound in nature, it may be difficult to determine what has been acquired at the workplace. The infectious agents responsible for occupationally related skin disease depend on the geographic location as well as on the field of work.

Viruses

Viral agents include herpex simplex, which may be transmitted from infected patients to health care workers. Physicians, nurses, medical students, dentists, and dental hygienists are at high risk. Clinically, a painful herpetic whitlow will arise several days after direct contact with an infectious source. Animal handlers are also at increased risk of contracting viral agents. Milker's nodules, caused by a paravaccinia virus, and cowpox, caused by *Cowpox bovis,* develop on the hands after contact with cattle. Orf, also caused by a paravaccinia virus, is transmitted by infected sheep and goats. Warts, caused by human papillomavirus (HPV), develop on the hands of meat handlers at sites of meat contact. Similarly, hand warts occur more frequently in fish handlers. HPV-7 is found almost exclusively in butchers and fish handlers, although other HPV types commonly cause warts in both of these groups.[39,40] Human parvovirus B19 infection, which causes erythema infectiosum (fifth disease) and may be associated with arthritis and fetal death, is an occupational risk factor for school and day-care personnel.[41]

Bacteria

Bacterial infections are promoted by heat, humidity, occlusion, and lack of hygiene; therefore, military personnel, explorers, tunnelers, and those working in hot, enclosed spaces are most susceptible.[42] Notably, pyogenic infections due to *Staphylococcus aureus* and *streptococci* group A may erupt clinically as impetigo, furuncles, paronychia, and abscesses.[43]

Animal handlers are at particular risk for other bacterial infections. Anthrax is caused by *Bacillus anthracis,* and lesions are localized on exposed body parts 2 to 3 days after inoculation. A red patch initially occurs, later becoming vesicular and pustular. At risk are people in direct contact with infected animals, such as veterinary workers, slaughterhouse employees, wool sorters, and farmers. High-risk individuals should receive vaccination and education about transmission.[44] Brucellosis, caused by *Brucella abortus, B. melitensis,* and *B. suis,* may also be acquired by contact with infected animals. A papulopustule with lymph node enlargement occurs most typically in veterinarians, slaughterhouse workers, meat packers, and laboratory technicians.[45] Tularemia, manifesting as an ulcer at the inoculation site, is caused by *Francisella tularensis*. Although recreational hunters are at greatest risk, the disease also affects veterinarians, farmers, butchers, foresters, and laboratory personnel. The most common animal carriers include rabbits, deer, squirrels, skunks, and muskrats.[45] Cat scratch disease, caused by *Afipia felis,* may be contracted in cat handlers or veterinarians. Clinically, a papule or nodule may develop at the scratch site, followed by the enlargement of regional lymph nodes.[45] Erysipeloid, caused by *Erysipelothrix rhusiopathiae,* infests fish, crabs, other shellfish, pigs, rabbits, and poultry. Human infection occurs through a break in the skin; fishermen, butchers, animal breeders, and cooks are at highest risk.[42] Glanders, manifesting as a papulopustular lesion which eventually ulcerates, occurs when *Pseudomonas mallei* gains entrance through the skin of persons handling horses or in contact with laboratory organisms.[43]

Mycobacterial infections may also be occupationally related. Cutaneous tuberculosis may be acquired by contact in pathologists, morgue attendants, surgeons, veterinarians, farmers, and butchers. Atypical mycobacterial infections are also transmitted through small breaks in the skin. *Mycobacterium marinum* is the most commonly acquired infection; high-risk persons include fish tank cleaners and Gulf of Mexico fishermen.[45] Rickettsial infections may be transmitted to soldiers, explorers, surveyors, and farmers through arthropod bites. Similarly, in many parts of the world erythema chronicum migrans, a characteristic of Lyme disease, may occur in outdoor workers after a tick bite.

Fungi

There are multiple occupationally related fungal infections. *Candida albicans* is the most common occupationally acquired fungal infection.[45] Paronychial candidal infection occurs in workers whose hands are constantly exposed to moisture. *Candida* infection commonly favors areas where skin surfaces are in apposition and is promoted by moist, warm work environments. Dermatophyte infections may be transmitted to medical and dental workers, farmers, and veterinarians. Tinea barbae and tinea manuum may present as inflammatory kerion celsi type, suppurative nodular, or superficial circinate lesions. The most common causes are *Trichophyton mentagrophytes, T. verrucosum, T. rubrum, T. violaceum,* and *Microsporum canis.*[43] Tinea capitis, caused by *T. tonsurans* or *M. audouini,* may be transmitted to barbers.[45]

Laboratory workers are at risk for deep mycotic infection by transcutaneous entry, typically through skin breaks. Reports of deep mycoses in laboratory workers have been noted with sporotrichosis, histoplasmosis, coccidioidomycosis, and blastomycosis.[45,46] Characteristically, the lesions are present at the site of inoculation. Sporotrichosis, caused by *Sporothrix schenckii,* may be transmitted by contact with timber, sphagnum moss, marsh hay, barberry bushes, and other plant material. The most frequently infected workers are gardeners, florists, greenhouse workers, and farm hands; however, all occupational groups in contact with vegetable material are at risk, such as chefs, pottery workers, and miners.[46] Animal bites from fish, snakes, birds, rodents, bats, dogs, and insects may also transmit the disease.[46] Erythema nodosum or erythema multiforme may be a manifestation of histoplasmosis. Workers involved in demolition of buildings and excavation for new construction are at risk, as well as those in contact with decaying trees, storm cellars, and topsoil. Farmers are at particularly high risk, as well as spelunkers, due to bat transmission of *Histoplasma capsulatum* in caves.[46] Coccicioidomycosis, caused by *Coccidioides imitis,* may appear clinically as localized lesions in sites of primary inoculation. Secondary erythema nodosum is frequent following respiratory exposure to this organism. This fungus also exists in soil and may be transmitted to archaeologists and farm workers; fruits, cotton, and vegetables may also be fungus laden.[46] Blastomycosis, caused by *Blastomyces dermatitidis,* has occurred after puncture or cutting wounds in laboratory and autopsy workers.[46] One cause of primary pulmonary inoculation occurred in a laboratory worker after inhaling a culture of *B. dermatitidis.*[46]

Parasites

Certain occupational groups, in association with particular geographic location, are vulnerable to parasitic infestations. Cutaneous larva migrans may be caused by *Ancyclostoma braziliense, A. duodenale,* or *Necator amcircanus.* Skin findings demonstrate thin, wandering, raised, pruritic lines and occasional scaling. Subtropical and tropical workers in contact with warm, moist soil or sand are also at risk, including agricultural laborers, sewer workers, ditch diggers, and lifeguards.[45] Swimmer's itch due to schistosomes causing urticaria is most likely to occur in skin divers, lifeguards, dock workers, and lake or pond workers.[45] Sea bather's eruption is frequent in southeast Florida divers and lifeguards. Scabies, especially Norwegian scabies, may be transmitted from patients to health care workers. Anal pruritus, caused by pinworms, is a risk to schoolteachers and child care workers.[42] Grain itch, a pruritic maculopapular eruption produced by mites, may affect dockers, cargo workers, transporters, millers, bakers, and grocers.[42] Similarly, various arthropod bites may cause primary reactions or pass disease such as Lyme disease in outdoor workers.

REACTIONS TO TEMPERATURE AND HUMIDITY

Heat and High Humidity

Miliaria is an inflammatory reaction to retained extravasated sweat resulting from sweat duct obstruction. It manifests as pinhead-sized papules and vesicles on the chest and back, as well as in the submammary, inguinal, and axillary folds. It is most common in workers exposed to heat and high humidity who sweat profusely.[3] Intertrigo occurs on opposing skin surfaces as a scaling, erythematous eruption. Again, workers exposed to heat and high humidity are at higher risk. Superimposed fungal infections may result, as discussed previously.

Low Humidity

Pruritus, xerosis, and eczema may result in workers exposed to low-humidity environments due to stratum corneum dehydration, noted at relative humidities of less than 60%.[47] Complaints occur more frequently in the winter, when warm, unhumidified air is vented into offices, more likely affecting those working near heating vents. Other workers at risk include those in airplanes, hospitals, hotels, and factories, as well as traveling salespeople in heated automobiles.[47]

SCLERODERMA

Scleroderma is characterized by fibrosis and degenerative changes in the skin and in some cases has been associated with a number of different occupational exposures. It is important to remember that scleroderma is also a generalized multisystemic disease involving the vasculature and internal organs. The skin findings in occupational scleroderma may be identical to the cutaneous sclerosis found in acrosclerosis and generalized cutaneous sclerosis, including Raynaud's phenomenon.[48]

Silica-induced scleroderma has been reported in underground goldminers, sand blasters, and workers in potteries and foundries.[49] Exposure is typically from inhalation of silica dust, and the length of exposure prior to development of symptoms is measured in years.[50] The features are clinically, serologically, and immunologically indistinguishable from those of patients with the idiopathic form of scleroderma; unfortunately, the lack of spontaneous remission is also characteristic.[48]

In the plastics industry, scleroderma-like changes have been noted in workers engaged in the polymerization of vinyl chloride due to inhalation or transcutaneous absorption of vinyl chloride. Clinically, vinyl chloride causes more localized fibrotic lesions, sparing the face and trunk. Raynaud's phenomenon and osteolysis in the distal phalangeal joints of the first three fingers, also called *acro-osteolysis,* may occur. Vinyl chloride disease is reversible, unlike silica-induced scleroderma.[51] Solvents and epoxy resins have also been implicated in occupationally induced, scleroderma-like changes.[52] Occupationally induced Raynaud's phenomenon may also be a sign of vibration-induced white finger disease (VWF). VWF is characterized by tingling, numbness, and blanching of the fingers provoked by exposure to cold and is caused by long-term use of hand-held vibratory tools.[53] VWF rarely progresses to scleroderma. In a recent report, three of the four cases of scleroderma associated with VWF had concomitant silica exposure.[54]

NAIL CHANGES

Occupationally induced nail changes have multiple manifestations and may have a traumatic, chemical, or infectious origin.[55] Manual laborers are especially prone to traumatic pathology, although most other occupations also have opportunities for traumatic nail injury.[56] Manifestations of nail trauma include subungual hematoma, splinter hemorrhage, leukonychia, onychodystrophy, onychochauxis, onycholysis, subungual hyperkeratosis, and traumatic pterygia.[55] Blue, brown, or yellow nail discoloration may occur from contact with bichromate, formaldehyde, amines, picric acid, nicotine, mercury, resorcin, vioform, or PCBs.[57] In addition to trauma, nail dystrophy may result from chemical exposures, namely, solvents, or from Raynaud's phenomenon, as seen in the vibratory trauma of jack hammer operators (VWF) and musicians.[58,59] Green nails, chronic paronychia, and associated dystrophy are most often associated with *Candida* and *Pseudomonas* species, which may occur in wet workers (bartenders, maintenance workers, kitchen workers).[3,55] Primary-inoculation tuberculosis in pathologists may also manifest in nail folds.[55] Arsenical poisoning may produce horizontal nail striations called *Mee's lines.*[59] Occupationally induced koilonychia or "spoon" nails may occur in workers exposed to motor oils[60] or organic solvents.

REFERENCES

1. Adams RM (ed): *Occupational Skin Disease,* ed 2. Philadelphia, WB Saunders, 1990.
2. Hogan DJ, Tanglertsampan C: The less common occupational dermatoses. *Occup Med: State of the Art Reviews* 7:385–401, 1992.
3. Taylor JS: Occupational dermatoses. In Alderman MH, Hanley MJ (eds): *Clinical Medicine for the Occupational Physician.* New York, Marcel Dekker, 1982, pp 299–344.
4. Zugerman C: Chloracne: Clinical manifestations and etiology. *Dermatol Clin* 8(1):209–213, 1990.
5. Taylor JS: Environmental chloracne: Update and overview. *Ann NY Acad Sci* 320:295–307, 1979.

REFERENCES

6. Crow KD, Puhvel SM: Choracne (halogen acne). In Maibach HI, Marzulli FN (eds): *Dermatotoxicology,* ed 4. New York, Hemisphere, 1991, pp 647–665.
7. Tindall JP: Chloracne and chloracnegens. *J Am Acad Dermatol* 13:539–558, 1985.
8. Crow KD: Chloracne. *Semin Dermatol* 1:305–314, 1982.
9. Gladen BC, Taylor JS, Wu YC, et al: Dermatological findings in children exposed transplacentally to heat-degraded polychlorinated biphenyls in Taiwan. *Br J Dermatol* 122:799–808, 1990.
10. Caputo R, Monti M, Ermacora E, et al: Cutaneous manifestations of tetrachlorodibenzo-*p*-dioxin in children and adolescents. *J Am Acad Dermatol* 19:812–819, 1988.
11. Assennato G, Cervino D, Emmet EA, et al: Follow-up of subjects who developed chloracne following TCDD exposure at Seveso. *Am J Indian Med* 16:119–125, 1989.
12. Silbergeld EK: Dioxin: A case study in chloracne. In Maibach HI, Marzulli FN (eds): *Dermatotoxicology,* ed 4. New York, Hemisphere, 1991, pp 667–686.
13. Bond GG, McLaren EA, Brenner FE, et al: Incidence of chloracne among chemical workers potentially exposed to chlorinated dioxins. *J Occup Med* 31:771–774, 1989.
14. Neuberger M, Landovoight W, Deratl F: Blood levels of 2,3,7,7-TCDD in chemical workers after chloracne and in comparison groups. *Int Arch Occup Environ Health* 63:325–327, 1991.
15. Leung HW, Murray FJ, Paustenbach DJ: A proposed occupational exposure limit for 2,3,7,8-TCDD. *Am Indust Hyg Assoc J* 49:466–474, 1988.
16. Lucier GW, Portier CJ, Gallo MA: Receptor mechanisms and dose–response models for the effects of dioxins. *Environ Health Perspect* 101:36–44, 1993.
17. Gellin GA: Pigment responses: Occupational disorders of pigmentation. In Maibach HI (ed): *Occupational and Industrial Medicine,* ed 2. Chicago, Yearbook, 1987, pp 134–141.
18. Nethercott J: Chemical agents associated with the development of skin cancer. Paper presented at the American Academy of Dermatology Conference, Environment and the Skin, Washington DC, October 1992.
19. Schwartz L, Tulipan L, Birmingham DJ: Occupational Diseases of the Skin. Philadelphia, Lea & Febiger, 1957, p 262.
20. Dickerson DB, Smith TH: Antimony, arsenic, and their compounds. In Zenz C (ed): *Occupational Medicine,* ed 2. Chicago, Year Book Medical, 1988, pp 509–516.
21. Birmingham DJ: Disorders due to chemical agents. In Fitzpatrick TB, Arendt KA, Clark WA, et al (eds): *Dermatology in General Medicine.* New York, McGraw-Hill, 1971, pp 1044–1061.
22. Stockinger HE: The metals. In Clayton GD, Clayton FE (eds): *Patty's Industrial Hygiene and Toxicology, Volume 2A,* ed 3. New York, Wiley, 1981, pp 1493–2060.
23. Mathias CG: Occupational dermatoses. *J Am Acad Dermatol* 19:1104–1107, 1988.
24. Fisher AA: Highlights of the AAD post-graduate course "Recent developments in contact dermatitis and occupational dermatology" sponsored by the AAD with the North American Contact Dermatitis Group San Diego, May 21–28. Part 1. *Cutis* 42:93–95, 1988.
25. Fisher AA: Vitiligo due to contactants. *Cutis* 17:431–432, 437, 438, 1976.
26. O'Malley MA, Mathias CG, Priddy M, et al: Occupational vitiligo due to unsuspected presence of phenolic antioxidant byproducts in commercial bulk rubber. *J Occup Med* 30:512–516, 1988.

27. Ross D: A look at skin cancer. *Occup Health (Lond)* 40:420–422, 1988.
28. Vickers CFH: Industrial carcinogenesis. *Br J Dermatol* 105(Suppl 21):57–61, 1981.
29. Weinstein AL, Howe HL, Burnett WS: Sentinel health surveillance: Skin cancer of the scrotum in New York State. *Am J Public Health* 79:1513–1515, 1989.
30. Jarvholm B, Easton D: Models for skin tumour risks in workers exposed to mineral oils. *Br J Cancer* 62:1039–1041, 1990.
31. Bates MN, Smith AH, Hopenhayn-Rich C: Arsenic ingestion and internal cancers: A review. *Am J Epidemiol* 135:462–476, 1992.
32. Borland RM, Hocking B, Godkin GA, et al: The impact of a skin cancer control education package for outdoor workers. *Med J Aust* 154:686–688, 1991.
33. Kelsey CA, Mettler FA: Flexible protective gloves: The emperor's new clothes. *Radiology* 174:275–276, 1990.
34. Cristofolini M, Francesch S, Tasin L, et al: Risk factors for cutaneous malignant melanoma in a northern Italian population. *Int J Cancer* 39:150–154, 1987.
35. Weiss J, Bertz J, Jung EG: Malignant melanoma in southern Germany: Different predictive value of risk factors for melanoma subtypes. *Dermatologica* 183:109–113, 1991.
36. McLaughlin JK, Malker HSR, Blot WJ: Malignant melanoma in the printing industry. *Am J Indian Med* 13:301–304, 1988.
37. Schneider JS, Moore DH, Sagebiel RW: Early diagnosis of cutaneous malignant melanoma at Lawrence Livermore National Laboratory. *Arch Dermatol* 126:767–769, 1990.
38. Schwartzbaum JA, Setzer W, Kupper LL: An exploratory analysis of the occupational correlates of large pigmented nevi at Lawrence Livermore National Laboratory. *J Occup Med* 32:605–611, 1990.
39. Jablonska S, Obalek S, Golebiowska A: Epidemiology of butcher's warts. *Arch Dermatol Res* 280:524–528, 1988.
40. Rudlinger R, Bunney MH, Grob R, et al: Warts in fish handlers. *Br J Dermatol* 120:375–381, 1989.
41. Gillespie SM, Cartter ML, Asch S, et al: Occupational risk of human parvovirus B19 infection for school and day-care personnel during an outbreak of erythema infectiosum. *JAMA* 263:2061–2065, 1990.
42. Wilkinson DS: Biologic causes of occupational dermatoses. In Maibach HI (ed): *Occupational and Industrial Medicine,* ed 2. Chicago, Year Book Medical, 1987, pp 56–74.
43. Meneghini CL: Occupational microbial dermatoses. In Maibach HI (ed): *Occupational and Industrial Medicine,* ed 2. Chicago, Year Book Medical, 1987, pp 75–87.
44. Anonymous: Human cutaneous anthrax—North Carolina, 1987. *MMWR* 37:413–414, 1988.
45. Adams RM: Physical and biologic causes of occupational skin disease. In Adams RM (ed): *Occupational Skin Disease.* New York, Grune & Stratton, 1983, pp 27–57.
46. Schwarz J, Kauffman CA: Occupational hazards from deep mycoses. *Arch Dermatol* 113:1270–1275, 1977.
47. Rycroft RJG: Low-humidity occupational dermatoses. *Dermatol Clin* 2:553–559, 1984.
48. Rustin MHA, Bull HA, Ziegler V, et al: Silica-associated systemic sclerosis is clinically, serologically, and immunologically indistinguishable from idiopathic systemic sclerosis. *Br J Dermatol* 123:725–734, 1990.

REFERENCES

49. Owens GR, Medsger TA: Systemic sclerosis secondary to occupational exposure. *Am J Med* 85:114–116, 1988.
50. Haustein UF, Ziegler V, Herrman K, et al: Silica induced scleroderma. *J Am Acad Dermatol* 22:444–448, 1990.
51. Zschunke E, Ziegler V, Uwe-Frithjof H: Occupationally induced connective tissue disorders. In Adams RM (ed): *Occupational Skin Disease,* ed 2. Philadelphia, WB Saunders, 1990, pp 176–178.
52. Straniero NR, Furst DE: Environmentally-induced systemic sclerosis-like illness. *Baillieres' Clin Rheumatol* 3:63–79, 1989.
53. Taylor JS: Vibration syndrome in industry: Dermatological viewpoint. *Am J Indian Med* 8:415–432, 1985.
54. Pelmear PL, Roos JO, Maehle WM: Occupationally-induced scleroderma. *J Occup Med* 34:20–25, 1992.
55. Scher RK: Occupational nail disorders. *Dermatol Clin* 6:27–33, 1988.
56. Positano RG, DeLauro TM, Berkowitz BJ: Nail changes secondary to environmental influences. *Clin Podiatr Med Surg* 6:417–429, 1989.
57. Fischbein A, Wolff MS, Lilis R, et al: Clinical findings among PCB-exposed capacitor manufacturing workers. *Ann NY Acad Sci* 320:703–715, 1979.
58. Helm TN, Taylor JS, Adams RM, et al: Skin problems of performing artists. *Am J Contact Dermatol* 4:27–32, 1993.
59. Gibbs RC, Leider M: Foot notes: A comprehensive, annotated, and partially illustrated table of conditions in, under, and around toe and finger nails. *J Dermatol Surg Oncol* 5:467–473, 1979.
60. Dawber R: Occupational koilonychia. *Br J Dermatol* 91(Suppl 10):11, 1974.

9

Treatment of Occupational Dermatitis

Joseph F. Fowler, Jr.

Occupational dermatitis almost always affects the hands primarily; therefore, all the difficulties inherent in treating hand eczema must be considered, along with specific workplace factors. Treatment may need to be more intensive or of greater duration than in nonoccupational settings. Not only medical factors but also socioeconomic considerations are important.

GENERAL PRINCIPLES OF TREATMENT

An accurate diagnosis is essential for proper treatment. This almost always means that patch testing must be done to evaluate possible allergens. Furthermore, it is helpful to have the patient explain in some detail the exact nature of his job. This is helpful in selecting proper patch allergens and allows an estimate of degree of irritant exposure. Material Safety Data Sheets, although not usually helpful in finding allergens, contain valuable information on the irritancy potential of workplace substances. It is also important to know what protective and treatment measures the patient has already tried. At times, self-treatment may be exacerbating the dermatitis rather than helping to cure it. Allergy to the active ingredients or excipients in anesthetics, antihistamines, topical corticosteroids, antifungals, or antibiotics may occur. Allergy may also occur to protective gloves. Some substances readily penetrate certain intact gloves and then are held against the skin, thereby exacerbating the problem.

BARRIER CREAMS

Many so-called barrier creams are marketed to industrial companies. Occasionally they may offer modest protection against injury from solvents or alkalis. While they are good in theory, in practice any barrier effect lasts only as long as the cream coats the skin. Wiping the hands, friction from gloves, and other sources remove the cream fairly rapidly. In fact, by applying a barrier cream to already irritated skin, further irritation and allergic sensitization to a component of the cream may occur. Propylene glycol and para-chloro-meta-xylenol, a preservative and an antiseptic, respectively, which are often found in barrier creams, are typical examples.[1]

The only proven instance of efficacy of a barrier cream applies to poison ivy, oak, and sumac. Orchard and colleagues have shown that Stokogard Cream (Stockhausen Skin Protection, Greensboro, NC), a compound of linoleic acid dimers, provides fairly good protection from *Rhus* allergy.[2] The cream apparently binds the resin and keeps it from penetrating the stratum corneum. Protection lasts for 6–8 hr, and then the cream and resin should be washed off. This cream may also protect against other plant allergens.[3] Another compound, called an *organoclay,* has been undergoing tests for *Rhus* protectivity and appears to be very promising.

PROTECTIVE GLOVES

Many types of gloves are available for occupational hand protection. Latex, nitrile, and neoprene are types of rubber gloves useful for various exposures. Vinyl gloves may offer an alternative for some rubber-sensitive individuals in certain settings. Certain gloves offer superior protection from a particular contactant, depending on the glove material and the nature of the exposure. Industrial glove manufacturers can provide lists of penetration times for various materials with each glove type (see Appendix 2). Organic solvents, for instance, are generally less able to penetrate nitrile rubber and plastic laminates than natural rubber or vinyl.

Two particular glove types deserve special mention. The 4-H glove (Safety 4 Company, Lyngby, Denmark) is a polyethylene laminate glove. Although quite thin and flexible, it offers superior resistance to a number of chemicals. Of particular interest to occupational dermatology are the allergens glyceryl thioglycolate and acrylates. The former causes frequent hand eczema in hairdressers. The latter may cause allergy in dental workers, some physicians, and chemical (plastics, oils) workers. Significant and often severe hand eczema is fairly common with these allergens. The 4-H glove effectively blocks contact of these items with the skin for reasonable periods of time. It may also be useful for protecting against epoxy resin.[3] The Tactyl-1 glove (Smart Practice, Phoenix, AZ) is a polystyrene glove that has the distensibility and feel of latex without containing any latex allergen.[4] With the significant increase in latex contact urticaria, especially among health care workers, this glove may be very useful. The protective benefits of this glove are similar to those of standard medical gloves, but the risk of latex reactions in patients or wearers is absent. Although expensive compared to latex gloves, this glove may allow a medical worker with latex allergy to continue in his or her occupation.

The use of cotton gloves underneath rubber or other protective gloves is helpful to absorb perspiration and reduce frictional irritation. Changing gloves frequently is important as well. Cotton gloves are not very effective in preventing sensitization and reactions to rubber glove allergens such as latex or accelerators contacting the skin. Rubber gloves with a fabric lining are of less benefit than plain gloves with cotton gloves underneath.

ANTIBIOTICS

Occasionally, systemic antibiotics may be useful in severe cases of hand eczema that have or may become secondarily infected. Erythromycin or a penicillin derivative such as dicloxacillin are usually effective. In addition, hand eczema in atopics may improve with systemic antibiotics that reduce the skin colonization by staphylococci. Topical antibiotics should usually be avoided because of the high rate of sensitization, at least to neomycin and bacitracin. Mupirocin ointment is less likely to sensitize but is expensive.

HAND WASHING

Frequent or prolonged hand washing should be avoided in both allergic and irritant hand eczema. Thorough rinsing is important even with mild soaps. Use of solvents to clean the hands, such as paint thinner or gasoline, should be strictly avoided. Fisher recommends bathing the hands in dilute Burrow's solution in the acute edematous stage of hand eczema.[5] It is advisable to remove rings when washing the hands to avoid trapping of soap and moisture under the rings. Use of emollients may help reduce the adherence of dirt and grease to the skin, thereby reducing the need for vigorous hand washing.

EMOLLIENTS

The ideal emollient would be nongreasy, easy to rub into the skin, unscented, free of sensitizing allergens, able to improve skin hydration, protective against further damage, and inexpensive. Since such a product does not exist, many varieties of skin creams and lotions attempt to fill the bill. Pure petrolatum is quite safe and economical, and may be used at certain times when the individual does not need to use the hands. It is too greasy, however, to be practical in working situations. Essentially the choice of an emollient is one of personal preference of the physician or patient. Products containing fragrances or other common allergens should be avoided. Recently, the alpha hydroxy acids have been suggested as ingredients in moisturizers that may be especially helpful in hydrating the skin. Lactic and glycolic acids are most commonly used. A drawback is that products containing these acids commonly burn or sting if applied to dermatitic skin. They may be more useful in preserving healthy skin than in treating already irritated skin. Glycerine is another ingredient that may increase the water-holding capacity of the skin.[6]

TREATMENT OF IRRITANT CONTACT DERMATITIS

The basic principle of treatment of irritant contact dermatitis (ICD) is the restoration of the normal cutaneous barrier function. Nearly always, either protection of the skin by gloves or other methods, or temporary removal from the causative environment, or both must be accomplished. Without pharmacologic intervention, this restoration may take weeks or even months to complete.

Lubrication and hydration of the skin with emollients, as noted above, is critical. Early on, low- to midpotency topical corticosteroids are helpful in reducing inflammation. Since the cell-mediated immune system is not the primary cause of the pathology, potent systemic topical corticosteroids are not usually of great benefit. Lubricating agents must not be greasy enough to interfere with functioning at work and at home. A simple compound that is well accepted is noted in Table 9-1A. This mixture is nongreasy and should be applied frequently (5–10 times daily). It may substitute for a nonprescription hand lotion. Once healing has been achieved, an over-the-counter emollient may be substituted if desired. The pain of fissures and cracks may be dramatically alleviated by applying a quick-curing acrylate glue (Super Glue) to the cracks. Care must be taken so that the fingers and hands do not become stuck together in the process of application. A cotton-tip applicator or toothpick is suggested. Another preparation that is inexpensive and tolerable to most patients is a mixture of equal parts triamcinolone 0.1% cream and oint-

TABLE 9-1 Preparations for Irritant Contact Dermatitis

A. Hydrocortisone, 1% (powder)
   Propylene glycol, 12 g
   Acid Mantle Cream q.s.a.d., 120 g
   Sig: Apply 5–10 times per day sparingly
   For fissures
   Apply a small amount of Super Glue to the fissure with an applicator or toothpick. Let dry thoroughly.
B. Triamcinolone 0.1% cream, 60 g
   Triamcinolone 0.1% ointment q.s.a.d., 120 g
   Sig: Apply sparingly as frequently as needed
   (Courtesy of C. G. T. Mathias)

ment. This is less greasy than the pure ointment but more moisturizing than the cream alone (personal communication, C. G. Toby Mathias, Cincinnati, OH).

TREATMENT OF ALLERGIC CONTACT DERMATITIS

In contrast to ICD, treatment of severe acute contact dermatitis (ACD) usually requires systemic corticosteroids. Oral prednisone, 40–60 mg/day or its equivalent, may be required. Tapering over 14–21 days, depending on the degree of dermatitis and the severity of exposure, is usual. Initially, potent topicals may be needed, but they usually should not be used beyond a few weeks. Subsequently, the compounds listed in Table 9-1 may be employed. In patients for whom compliance may be problematic, intramuscular corticosteroids such as triamcinolone or methylprednisolone may be useful. In addition, the prolonged effect of intramuscular therapy may help by allowing the skin time to heal and become more resistant to further damage. Obviously without allergen avoidance, no amount of treatment will suffice.

Antihistamines are of some benefit in minimizing pruritus. Their sedating effects may be desirable as well in some cases. Terfenadine and other nonsedating antihistamines are probably not as effective for reducing pruritus as other antihistamines like hydroxyzine and cyproheptadene. For chronic dermatitis, adding anti-inflammatory agents or keratolytics may be helpful in avoiding the need for continuous use of potent topical steroids (Table 9-2A). An antipruritic topical mixture is given in Table 9-2B.

Injection of dilute (4–7 mg/mc) triamcinolone acetonide directly into dermatitic areas may sometimes produce a prolonged response. However, this tends to be much more painful than on most other body areas, which may limit patient acceptance. Nevertheless, when it is inadvisable to use systemic corticosteroids, this may be a very successful therapy.

Some cases of ACD develop into a chronic smoldering dermatitis. This

TABLE 9-2 Useful Mixtures for Chronic Contact Dermatitis

A. Salicylic acid, 2%
   Liquor carbonis detergens, 2%
   Betamethasone Valerate Cream, 60 g
   Velvachol q.s.a.d., 180 g
   Sig: Apply t.i.d. to affected areas
   (Courtesy of Dr. L. G. Owen, Louisville, KY)

B. 1/4% menthol
   1/4% phenol
   Betametasone Dipropionate Lotion, 60 cc
   Aqua Glycolic Lotion q.s.a.d., 8 oz
   Sig: Apply to itchy areas b.i.d. to q.i.d.

has been particularly recognized in the case of chromate hand dermatitis. At other times allergen avoidance is difficult—for instance, with formaldehyde or nickel allergy. In such chronic cases, psoralen plus ultraviolet A (PUVA) therapy is sometimes useful. The psoralen may be administered topically in liquid or ointment form or may be given systemically. Topical treatment with methoxypsoralen avoids systemic side effects but may be more likely to cause a local burn. Oral therapy may be more effective, with less chance of burning. Usually 2 or 3 treatments per week are used until remission results (typically, 20–25 treatments). Maintenance therapy can then proceed at weekly (or less frequent) intervals.

Superficial x-rays (Grenz rays) are occasionally still used for chronic dermatitis, especially of the hands. One treatment of 200 rads may provide relief for up to a month. Because the radiation penetrates minimally, serious sequelae such as skin cancer are unlikely. Both PUVA and grenz rays may reduce the need for systemic corticosteroid treatment.

NOVEL THERAPIES FOR HAND ECZEMA

Disulfiram for Nickel Allergy

Although nickel allergy, like most types of ACD, usually manifests as dermatitis at the site of contact, hand eczema may occur due to systemic nickel ingestion in food. Disulfiram chelates nickel ions in vivo, allowing the excretion of nickel in urine and stool.[7] Accordingly, it has been found helpful in some cases of nickel allergic hand eczema that do not respond to conventional treatments.[8,9] A dose of 250 mg/d may be employed for 4–6 weeks. Often an initial flare of dermatitis may occur from mobilization of nickel. If beneficial effects are seen, the drug may be continued as needed. Absolute alcohol avoidance is necessary, since the disulfiram–alcohol interaction may cause severe systemic symptoms. Liver function tests should be monitored.

Dietary Modification

In addition to nickel, some investigators believe that other metals (cobalt and chromate) and spices or flavorings (e.g., Balsam of Peru–related substances) may exacerbate allergic dermatitis when ingested.[10–12] Diet modification to reduce the intake of these items is reportedly helpful in some cases.

Dapsone

Dapsone (100 mg/day) was reported to improve hand eczema in five cement workers with chromate allergy. Reduction in the level of toxic superoxide radicals in tissue was postulated to be the reason for improvement.[13]

Chromate Barrier Cream

Romaguera and colleagues reported beneficial results in some chromate-sensitive construction workers using a barrier cream composed of silicone, tartaric acid, glycine, and other ingredients.[14] The tartaric acid and glycine apparently chelate chromate and reduce chrome VI to chrome III, which is less allergenic.

SUMMARY

Treatment of hand eczema depends first on an accurate diagnosis and avoidance of allergens if indicated. Protective and preventive measures, such as wearing gloves or protective clothing and short-term changes in job exposure, are often needed. Protective barrier creams are helpful only in selected situations. Topical emollients and corticosteroid agents are frequently used. Systemic corticosteroids may be necessary for allergic dermatitis. Occasionally, ultraviolet light or superficial x-rays may be used in recalcitrant cases.

REFERENCES

1. Mackey S, Marks J: Dermatitis in machinists: A retrospective study. *Am J Contact Dermatitis* 4:22–26, 1993.
2. Orchard S, Fellman JH, Storrs FJ: Poison ivy/oak dermatitis. Use of polyamine salts of a linolein acid dimer for topical prophylaxis. *Arch Dermatol* 122:783–789, 1986.
3. McClain DC, Storrs FJ: Protective effect of both a barrier cream and a polyethylene laminate glove against epoxy resin, glyceryl monothioglycolate, frullania, and tansy. *Am J Contact Dermatitis* 13:201–205, 1992.
4. Hamann CP: Natural rubber latex protein sensitivity in review. *Am J Contact Dermatitis* 4:4–21, 1993.
5. Fisher AA, *Contact Dermatitis*, ed 3. Philadelphia, Lea & Febiger, 1984, pp 269–273.
6. Jackson BM: Moisturizers. What's in them? How do they work? *Am J Contact Dermatitis* 3:162–168, 1992.
7. Menne T, Kaaber K: Treatment of pompholyx due to nickel allergy with chelating agents. *Contact Dermatitis* 4:289–292, 1978.
8. Fowler JF: Disulfiram is effective for nickel allergic hand eczema. *Am J Contact Dermatitis* 3:175–178, 1992.
9. Kaaber K, Menne T, Hougaard P: Treatment of nickel dermatitis with Antabuse: Double-blind study. *Contact Dermatitis* 9:297–300, 1983.
10. Fowler J: Allergic contact dermatitis to metals. *Am J Contact Dermatitis* 1:212–223, 1990.

REFERENCES

11. Kaaber K, Veien N: Chromate ingestion in chronic chromate dermatitis. *Contact Dermatitis* 4:119–122, 1978.
12. Klaschka F, Ring J: Systemically induced (hematogenous) contact eczema. *Semin Dermatol* 9:210–215, 1990.
13. Miyachi Y, Uchida K, Komura J, et al: Autooxidative damage in cement dermatitis. *Arch Dermatol* 121:277–288, 1985.
14. Romaguera C, Grimalt F, Vilaplana J, et al: Formulation of a barrier cream against chromate. *Contact Dermatitis* 12:49–52, 1985.

10

Nondermatologic Aspects of Occupational Dermatology

Christopher J. Dannaker

INTRODUCTION

This chapter reviews issues in occupational dermatology of concern to clinical dermatologists. The topics covered include evaluating workers for occupationally related dermatoses, appropriate working and consulting relationships with workers and management, the protocol for undertaking plant tours, spot tests for chemicals, writing medical reports, identifying and correcting problems in the workplace environment, understanding industrial hygiene, governmental agencies and how they affect the workplace environment, interacting with worker's compensation insurance carriers and other potential problems and concerns of physicians.

Occupational skin diseases are the most reported occupational diseases in the United States. Such skin diseases account for approximately 30–40% of *all* occupational diseases. Due to underreporting, their true incidence may be as much as 10 to 50 times greater than the incidence estimated from government statistics.

Several industries have reported particularly high incidences of occupational skin disease. Those highlighted industries are useful for the dermatologist to note (Table 10-1).

TABLE 10-1 Industries with a High Incidence of Occupational Skin Disease

Industry	Incidence rate (per 1000 employees)
Leather tanning and fishing	21.2
Poultry dressing plants	16.4
Adhesives and sealants	12.6
Boat building and repairing	11.1
Fresh or frozen fish packaging	10.6
Poultry and egg processing	10.2
Abrasive products	9.3
Landscape and horticultural services	9.2
Farm labor and management services	8.9
Forestry services	8.9
Sanitation goods	8.4
Plating and polishing	8.3
Chemical preparations	8.3

Adapted from US Department of Labor, Report of the Advisory Committee on Cutaneous Hazards (1978).[2]

DECIDING IF DERMATITIS IS OCCUPATIONAL

There is no clinical or histologic sine qua non for diagnosing eczematous dermatitis resulting from occupational exposures. Therefore, the physician evaluating working populations is required to synthesize information from various sources, including the physical examination, workplace surveys, epidemiologic evidence, toxicology of chemical exposures, and industrial hygiene information.

After consideration of the findings, the physician detective is required to arrive at a reasonable probability for occupational causation, utilizing powers of deduction based on historical and physical evidence.

Histories must by necessity be extensive (Table 10-2).

Legal definitions of occupational dermatitis vary by country and, in the United States, from state to state. In some states, a skin disease may be considered occupational if it is only 1% caused or aggravated by workplace exposures. In other states, causation is accepted only if evidence of 50% or greater aggravation is present.

ASKING THE RIGHT QUESTIONS*

Fundamental questions should be kept in mind when the physician is considering the possibility of occupational causation for patient's dermatitis.[1]

*This section is an adaptation, with permission, from Reference 1.

Table 10-2 General Workup of a Possible Occupationally Related Disorder

I. A clue in the patient's history leads to the suspicion of a health complaint involving the work environment.
   A. Take a *history of the symptoms.*
   B. Temporal relationship between work and onset of the symptoms: do symptoms worsen during work and improve during weekends/vacations?
   C. Take a *relevant* occupational history.
   D. Important information for a case
      1. Company name.
      2. Name and telephone number of union and shop steward.
      3. Name of referring doctor and address.
      4. Name of lawyer and address if applicable.
      5. Name of plant's doctor, registered nurse, or industrial hygienist.
   E. Additional history to include: family history, past medical history, review of systems, medications; social history to include: educational level, use of cigarettes, alcohol, recreational drugs, spouse's job and exposures, hobbies.
II. Complete the occupational history.
   A. Home environment: living near factories or chemical waste dumps, indoor air pollution, use of toxic cleaners or hobby chemicals, etc.
   B. Complete occupational history
      1. Start in high school and work forward. Include even brief jobs which could have involved chemical exposures.
      2. Summer and part-time jobs, military service.
      3. Obtain the name of each company worked for, duties, and chemicals involved.
         a. What specific jobs/work processes did the patient do in a given day/week? Length of shift?
         b. What was the company's finished product?
         c. Did any other coworkers have similar problems?
         d. Is there any correlation between changes in duties or plant processes and the onset of symptoms?
         e. What chemicals, metals, solvents, or gases were used by the patient or coworkers? Quantities used? Any odors present?
         f. Were any physical stressors present (noise, extremes of heat or cold, humidity, vibration)?
         g. Protection (general work hygiene, personal protective devices such as gloves, respirators, aprons, showers, bathroom facilities).
         h. Job satisfaction/level of stress.
         i. Was OSHA or NIOSH ever called in? Were any citations given?

Source: Adapted from Kelley Ann Brix M.D., M.P.H., unpublished document.

Is There a Temporal Association between Exposure and the Onset of Eczematous Dermatitis?

The first or increased exposure to a physical or chemical hazard should, of course, precede the onset of dermatitis.

It is necessary to appreciate the existence of competing irritants at home in leisure-time activities. Irritants may be tolerated initially, but once the skin's tolerance is exhausted, clinical dermatitis may develop. Latency periods for acquisition of allergic contact dermatitis may span days or decades. Variables include the potency of an allergen, the magnitude of exposure, and host factors such as atopy and altered epidermal barrier.

Contact urticaria may manifest as subclinical dermatitis or stinging. Nondermatologic symptoms such as asthma and chronic sinusitis may also be a manifestation of the contact urticaria syndrome. Refractory periods, in which contact with a contact urticant may temporarily fail to elicit an allergic response, are possible and should not dissuade the knowledgeable physician from suspecting the presence of contact urticaria.

Is the Clinical Appearance that of an Eczematous Dermatitis?

Dermatologic disorders are common to the general populace and are expected to occur with equal frequency among the working population. Diseases such as psoriasis and porphyria cutanea tarda may mimic occupational dermatitis. Conversely, chronic contact dermatitis may mimic psoriasis or lichen simplex chronicus. Nummular dermatitis may occur due to secondary spread of a work-related allergen through transfer via the hands. Airborne allergic contact dermatitis may at first appear to be an unrelated photosensitivity disorder.

Are There Workplace Exposures to Known or Suspected Causes of Irritant or Allergic Contact Dermatitis?

Complete information concerning the toxicologic hazards at work should be reviewed by the physician. In the United States, Material Safety Data Sheets (MSDSs) should be on file in the workplace for any chemicals classified as hazardous. Employees, their union representative, and an employee's physician have a legal right, through enactment of federal Right-To-Know law, to obtain copies of these documents.

Is the Location of the Dermatitis Consistent with the Distribution of the Cutaneous Exposure?

Usually, dermatitis is expected to be maximal over areas of greatest skin exposure. Exceptions to this rule also occur. Inoculation of a contact allergen may occur by touching the eyelids, face, or genitals with contaminated hands. Dermatitis may be severe due to the increased skin permeability of these areas.

Do the Patch Tests or Immediate Skin Tests Identify a Probable Causal Agent?

A thorough history and allergy patch testing are necessary to answer this question adequately.

Are There Nonoccupational Sources of Exposure to Allergens or Irritants?

Complete patch testing and immediate skin testing, when indicated, are usually necessary to identify home and hobby chemical allergens that may contribute to a case of occupational allergy.

Does the Dermatitis Improve Away from Work, and Does Reexposure Result in Flaring?

One week away from work should usually result in some improvement. Persistence may occur if the dermatitis is severe and has been untreated for a prolonged period, when home sources of allergens or irritants are present, and when endogenous sources of dermatitis such as atopy are contributing factors.

LEGAL CASES REQUIRE APPORTIONMENT OF BLAME

When a legal case is evaluated, the following points should be considered:

1. *To what extent is the person's constitution a part of the present dermatitis?* For example, persons with a history of atopic eczema are more prone to develop irritant dermatitis. The relationship, if any, of personal histories such as hay fever and asthma, or simply a family history of atopic diatheses, to a patient's susceptibility to dermatitis is less clear.
2. *Previous dermatologic conditions* may become worse through work. A patient with preexisting psoriasis may develop additional lesions due to Koebnerization by occupational irritant dermatitis or allergic contact dermatitis. Documentation for legal purposes becomes primary and may require examination of previous physician treatment records, in addition to taking a thorough history.
3. *Secondary contact allergies* such as to rubber accelerators in gloves worn at home, over-the-counter topical medications, and prescription medications may be causal in perpetuating dermatitis.
4. *A preexisting contact allergy* may result in occupational dermatitis from workplace exposures. For example, nickel allergy acquired from costume jewelry may provoke hand dermatitis in the workplace due to handling of nickel-plated objects such as tools.
5. *An allergic or irritant dermatitis originating at work* may be perpetuated by involuntary contact away from work. This is especially problematic when ubiquitous allergens such as chromate or formaldehyde are involved. If sensitization to the allergen occurred while working, allergic contact dermatitis resulting from nonoccupational exposure is in part occupational.

THE WORKPLACE SURVEY—LEAVING THE MEDICAL OFFICE ENVIRONMENT

Workplace examinations may be required when the results of office evaluation and patch testing are inconclusive. The physician's time is valuable, making excursions away from the office the exception. Still, workplace visits for those practitioners concerned with occupational diseases are occasionally necessary.

The survey should begin with an appointment made through the plant or personnel manager or representatives of the medical department. The requesting department may want to speak with the physician regarding his interpretation of the disease outbreak. Although bias may be apparent, any suggestions should be noted. Physicians are reminded that a conclusion should not be reached or a position stated until all relevant information gathered during the visit has been reviewed. Management may be understandably anxious, but again, conclusions are best delayed until the physician has had the opportunity to evaluate all information impartially.

The industrial hygienist, plant physician or nurse, shop steward, and other personnel may be able to give details on the incidence of past outbreaks of dermatitis. A discussion before the walk-through survey regarding the manufacturing process, materials used, chemical composition of materials, and raw chemical supplies will be helpful in understanding the manufacturing process as the dermatologist surveys the plant.

A worker may on occasion react to traces of an allergen from the work environment such as contaminants or by-products of the industrial process. The use of *spot tests to detect a chemical allergen* may be helpful in these circumstances. Many of these tests can be performed with a minimum of time and effort. Such tests are available for formaldehyde (Lutidine test), nickel (dimethylglyoxime), chromium (diphenylcarbazide), and epoxy resin (thin layer chromatography).[3]

The guide is usually chosen with regard to knowledge of the plant processes and may not necessarily be the plant physician. The industrial hygienist may be particularly helpful in regard to handling procedures, waste disposal, biologic hazards, engineering controls of chemical hazards, and use of personal protective devices such as gloves and respirators. Wash, break, and locker rooms should not be neglected. The various soaps and cleansing agents available should be noted.

During the survey, individual workers may be questioned only with the permission of the host guide. Questions should be factual; the workers' impressions or beliefs should not be asked for or mentioned.

When the outbreak of dermatitis affects a significant number of workers, the physician may be asked, or may ask, to interview and/or examine workers with dermatitis at work. Symptomatic workers must consent to such an examination; most are typically anxious to cooperate.

A *final report* must be submitted in a timely manner. The report should include epidemiologic information such as the number of workers exposed and affected, age, sex, and basic demographic information. Potential workplace chemical exposures should be identified and their skin and systemic toxicity discussed. The conclusions should also make note of suggested corrective measures (see below). The workers examined will often have more than one dermatologic problem, some perhaps not work related. In the report summary, worker examinations can be listed separately and anonymously, giving the diagnosis for each.

MAKING THE DIFFERENCE—INSTITUTING CORRECTIVE ACTIONS

The control of an outbreak of occupational dermatitis may include industrial hygiene measures. Whenever possible, substitution of another product for the offensive chemical(s) is preferred. When, for example, an allergic contact dermatitis is present, it is preferable to keep the employee working at the same job by changing to a substitute chemical. This strategy usually has less economic impact on the worker than does a change in job position.

Engineering changes should be considered a secondary means of controlling occupational dermatitis. These may include changes in ventilation (airborne contact dermatitis), enclosure, or isolation of an industrial process.

Administrative changes such as limiting a worker's exposure time, establishing prohibited areas, training in desired practices, and other work practice changes can also be considered.

The least preferable strategy is the use of personal protective devices. This mechanism for control of a hazard depends on the employee's compliance. Devices such as gloves and respirators may be cumbersome, reduce job efficiency, and lower morale. All these factors have an effect on compliance. Devices such as gloves may pose a hazard, such as when working near moving machinery or when secondary allergic sensitization to the protective device itself results (i.e., glove dermatitis).

MAINTAINING CREDIBILITY IN THE WORKPLACE

Understanding industrial hygiene terminology is helpful for any physician involved in plant surveys and evaluation of working individuals. The MSDS (see the section "Asking the Right Questions") is a valuable but limited resource for chemical information. The MSDSs for all chemicals considered hazardous are required to be on file at the workplace and available at the worker's request. Although recent improvements in these information sheets (Figure 10-1) have occurred, chemical information is often outdated and incomplete.

The manufacturing company's telephone number is listed on the MSDS and enables one to contact a knowledgeable party. Note that the MSDS must list only hazardous chemicals. Contact allergens, which may be trace additives, are usually not considered hazardous and therefore are often omitted from MSDSs. Therefore, when a reaction to a chemical such as a preservative or fragrance is suspected, the manufacturer must be queried directly and the MSDS not relied on to provide complete chemical information.

Sources of toxicologic information include computerized databases (Toxline, Medline, Grateful Med) and available toxicology texts. Not to be overlooked is information provided by the patient, who can be asked to write down trade names and manufacturers' names and to obtain labels from containers. The company or union may be telephoned. Most major chemical manufacturers have consumer or toxicology hotlines. For the practicing dermatologist, the article by Cohen should be reviewed when seeking information resources related to occupational dermatology.[4]

Threshold limit values (TLVs) are suggested maximal exposures to potentially hazardous chemicals and physical agents such as lasers or microwaves. These standards are used by industrial hygienists and usually refer to airborne, respirable concentrations of chemicals. A booklet of TLVs is published annually by the American Conference of Governmental Hygienists (ACGIH), a nongovernmental agency.

TLV values originated in 1970, when the Occupational Safety and Health Act (OSHA) was promulgated. All ACGIH values at that time were adopted as law and renamed *permissible exposure limits (PELs)*. The governmental OSHA PELs have not been updated significantly since 1970, and few new chemicals have been added. Therefore, the annually updated ACGIH TLVs usually provide the most recent and stringent values for hazardous workplace exposures.[5]

The ACGIH TLV booklet has a "skin" notation for some substances. This does not refer to a chemical's ability to induce irritation or allergy, but rather to its potential to cause human toxicity through cutaneous absorption (skin, mucous membranes, and eyes). This may be due to direct cutaneous or vapor exposures. Organophosphate pesticides such as Malathion are one example (Figure 10-2).

A quick reference guide also published by the ACGIH compares values for chemical and physical agent exposures of the ACGIH TLVs, OSHA PELs, National Institute for Occupational Safety and Health Recommended Exposure Limits (RELs), and Deutsche Forschungsgemeinschaft (DFG) German values[6] (Figure 10-3).

The ACGIH warns, "These limits are intended for use in the practice of industrial hygiene as guidelines or recommendations in the control of potential health hazards. . . . They should not be used by anyone untrained in the discipline of industrial hygiene."[5] Therefore, TLVs must be considered as recommendations only. A complete understanding of the nature of exposure (continuous, intermittent, spiking), individual factors in susceptibility (smoking, pregnancy, atopy), and the toxicity of the chemical involved (carcinogen, irritant, allergen, acute or chronic toxin) must all be considered prior to recommending safe exposure levels for a working population.

Regulatory and other governmental agencies must necessarily be understood when one enters the arena of occupationally related disease evaluation or treatment. The passage of the OSHA Act of 1970 created the *Occupational Safety and Health Administration (OSHA)*. This is the enforcement arm of the government concerned with occupational safety. OSHA standards for workplace chemical exposures are law. The *National Institute for Occupational*

☆ STAR
STUCCO PRODUCTS

MATERIAL SAFETY DATA SHEET

SECTION I—MATERIAL IDENTIFICATION

Product Name: Star Exterior Stucco

Manufactures Name: Star Stucco Products, Inc.

Address: 1815 E. Home Ave., Fresno, CA 93703

Emergency Telephone Number: (209) 233-4646

Date of Preparation: January 1, 1991

SECTION II—HAZARDOUS INGREDIENTS

Hazardous Components	CAS Numbers	OSHA PEL	ACGIH TLV MG/M3	Other
	12168-85-3	5	5	---
	10034-77-2	5	5	---
	14808-60-7	0.1	0.1	---
	12042-78-3	5	5	---
	12068-35-8	5	5	---
	1305-62-0	5	5	---
	130-97-1	5	5	---

SECTION III—PHYSICAL PROPERTIES

Solubility in Water: Slight

Appearance and Odor: Any color; no odor

The following properties are not applicable: Specific Gravity, Boiling Point, Vapor Pressure, Vapor Density, Melting Point, Evaporation Rate.

SECTION IV—FIRE AND EXPLOSION DATA

Noncombustible and not explosive.

SECTION V—REACTIVITY DATA

Stable, keep dry until used to preserve product utility.

Is not incompatible with other materials, will not decompose into hazardous byproducts and will not polymerize.

SECTION VI—SPILL PROCEDURES

If spilled, use dry cleanup methods that do not disperse the dust into the air. Avoid breathing the dust. Emergency procedures are not required.

Small amounts of material can be disposed of as common waste or returned to the container for later use if it is not contaminated.

Figure 10-1 Sample Material Data Safety Sheet.

SECTION VII—HEALTH HAZARD DATA

Classified as a nuisance dust by OSHA, MSHA and ACGIH. As such, the TLV is 5mg/m3 for respirable dust and 10mg/m3 for total dust. Not known to cause cancer. Exposure can affect the skin, the eyes and mucous membranes. Materials may become hazardous if particles are broken down to the respiratory size range and if these particles are inhaled. No adverse health effects were seen in animals after ingestion of the materials. The products, as shipped, contain no particles in the respirable size range. However, during shipping, handling, or use, the sand particles may be broken down to the respiratory size range that may be inhaled. These dusts are hazardous to the respiratory system because of the presence of free quartz.

ACUTE EXPOSURE: Can dry the skin and cause alkali burns. Dust can irritate the eyes and upper respiratory system. Toxic effects noted in animals include, for acute exposures, alveolar damage with pulmonary edema. In chronic exposure tests, a fibrosis was noted.

CHRONIC EXPOSURE: Dust can cause inflammation of the lining tissue of the interior of the nose and inflammation of the cornea. Hypersensitive individuals may develop an allergic dermatitis. Over exposure to inhaled quartz dusts may lead to chronic fibrotic lung disease known as Silicosis, a form of disabling, progressive and sometimes fatal pulmonary fibrosis characterized by the presence of typical nodulations in the lungs. Characteristic X-ray changes are noted. There are no reports of people becoming sensitized to sand. People with pre-existing lung diseases may have increased susceptibility to the health effects of respirable dusts.

EMERGENCY FIRST AID PROCEDURES: Irrigate eyes immediately and repeatedly with water (15 minutes minimum) and get prompt medical attention. Wash exposed skin areas with soap and water. Apply sterile dressings. If ingested, consult physician immediately. Drink water.

WARNING: This product contains one or more chemicals known to the state of California to cause cancer or birth defects or other reproductive harm.

SECTION VIII—SPECIAL PROTECTION

In dusty environments, the use of an OSHA, MSHA or NIOSH approved respirator and tight fitting goggles is recommended.

Local exhaust can be used, if necessary, to control airborne dust levels. The use of barrier creams or impervious gloves, boots and clothing to protect the skin from contact is recommended. Following work, workers should shower with soap and water. Precautions must be observed because burns occur with little warning - little heat is sensed.

Figure 10-1. (Continued)

Safety and Health (NIOSH) is the governmental research oganization concerned with control and research. NIOSH recommends safety and health standards based on its research findings, but these standards are not law unless promulgated by OSHA. The *Environmental Protection Agency (EPA)* is responsible for air and water quality and for most environmental problems. The EPA, for example, by authority of the Federal Insecticide, Fungicide and Rodenticide Act (FIFRA), regulates the use and effects of pesticides on agricultural workers and residual food levels.[7]

		ADOPTED VALUES			
		TWA		STEL	
Substance	[CAS #]	ppm[a]	mg/m[3b]	ppm[a]	mg/m[3b]
Isopropyl acetate [108-21-4] (1976)		250	1040	310	1290
Isopropyl alcohol [67-63-0] (1976)		400	983	500	1230
Isopropylamine [75-31-0] (1976)		5	12	10	24
N-Isopropylaniline [768-52-5]—Skin (1986)		2	11	—	—
Isopropyl ether [108-20-3] (1976)		250	1040	310	1300
• Isopropyl glycidyl ether (IGE) [4016-14-2] (1976)		50	238	75	356
Kaolin [1332-58-7] (1992)		—	2 (j)	—	—
Ketene [463-51-4] (1976)		0.5	0.86	1.5	2.6
‡◄••Lead [7439-92-1], inorg. dusts & fumes, as Pb (1986)		—	(0.15)	—	—
Lead arsenate [7784-40-9], as Pb₃(AsO₄)₂ (1985)		—	0.15	—	—
•■ Lead chromate [7758-97-6], as Pb (1991)		—	0.05, A2	—	—
as Cr (1991)		—	0.012, A2	—	—
Limestone, see Calcium carbonate					
■ Lindane [58-89-9]—Skin (1986)		—	0.5	—	—
Lithium hydride [7580-67-8] (1977)		—	0.025	—	—
L.P.G. (Liquified petroleum gas) [68476-85-7] (1987)		1000	1800	—	—
Magnesite [546-93-0] (1986)		—	10(e)	—	—
Magnesium oxide fume [1309-48-4] (1977)		—	10	—	—
◄ Malathion [121-75-5]— Skin (1977)		—	10	—	—
Maleic anhydride [108-31-6] (1977)		0.25	1.0	—	—
‡ Manganese [7439-96-5], as Mn					
‡•Dust & compounds (1988)—		--	(5)	—	—
‡ Fume (1979)		—	(1)	—	(3)
Manganese cyclopentadienyl tricarbonyl [12079-65-1], as Mn—Skin (1986)		—	0.1	—	—
Marble, see Calcium carbonate					
‡◄ Mercury [7439-97-6], as Hg—Skin					
Alkyl compounds (1980)		—	0.01	—	0.03
‡All forms except alkyl Vapor (1982)		—	(0.05)	—	—
‡•Aryl & inorganic compounds (1982)		—	(0.1)	—	—
• Mesityl oxide [141-79-7] (1981)		15	60	25	100
Methacrylic acid [79-41-4] (1981)		20	70	—	—
Methane [74-82-8] (1981)		—(c)	—	—	—
Methanethiol, see Methyl mercaptan					

Figure 10-2. Sample page from the ACGIH TLV booklet. Note "skin" notation for chemical Malathion. See text for explanation.

SUBSTANCE	ACGIH TLVs				OSHA PELs				NIOSH RELs				DFG MAKs		PEAK	CARCINOGEN
CAS #	TWA ppm	mg/m³	STEL/CEIL(C) ppm	mg/m³	TWA ppm	mg/m³	STEL/CEIL(C) ppm	mg/m³	TWA ppm	mg/m³	STEL/CEIL(C) ppm	mg/m³	TWA ppm	mg/m³		
Lindane (γ-Hexachloro-cyclohexane) 58-89-9		0.5		Skin		0.5		Skin		0.5		Skin		0.5	III	EPA-B2 (mixture with α & β) IARC-2B NTP-2
Lithium hydride 7580-67-8		0.025				0.025				0.025				0.025 (G),(H)		
L.P.G. (Liquified petroleum gas) 68476-85-7	1000	1800		(e)	1000	1800			1000	1800				(G)		
Magnesite 546-93-0		10				15*; 5** *Total dust **Respirable fraction				10*; 5** *Total dust **Respirable fraction						
Magnesium oxide 1309-48-4														6 (F)		
Magnesium oxide fume 1309-48-4		10				10* [15*] *Total particulate								6 (F)	II.1	
Malathion 121-75-5		10		Skin; (q)		10* [15*] Skin; *Total dust				10		Skin		15 (D),(G)		IARC-3
Maleic anhydride 108-31-6	0.25	1.0			0.25	1			0.25	1			0.1	0.4 (C),(S)	I	
Malononitrile 109-77-3									3	8						

OCCUPATIONAL EXPOSURE VALUES

Figure 10-3. Reference guide published by the ACGIH comparing ACGIH, OSHA, NIOSH, and DFG recommended safe exposures to potentially toxic chemicals.

123

REPORTING TO BIG BROTHER—THE INSURANCE ADJUSTER

Most medical-legal reports require the physician to render an opinion as to whether there is a connection between the occupation and the patient's dermatitis. Apportionment is often an important issue. To what degree do preexisting medical conditions contribute to the patient's dermatologic illness? In some countries, if only 1% of the patient's dermatologic illness is due to the occupation, then medical care for this illness becomes the responsibility of the worker's compensation insurance company. (See "Deciding if Dermatitis Is Occupational" p 113). The American Medical Association's *Guides to the Evaluation of Permanent Impairment* may assist the physician in making such a medical-legal assessment.

A sample template for occupational dermatology reports is provided by Adams[8] (Figure 10-4).

Name ______________________ Date ______________
Address ______________________ Age __________ Sex __________
Home phone __________ Soc.sec.no. __________ Referred by __________
Current employer (name and address) ______________________
__________ Job title at present ______________________
Employer at onset of injury (name and address) ______________________
____
Date employed ______________ Date terminated ______________
Job title at onset of injury ______________ Date ______________
Insurance carrier (name and address) ______________________
____

Present Illness

Date of onset ______________ Dates of disability ______________
Location at onset ______________________
Patient's description ______________________
____
____
____
Time off work (incl. vacations)? ______________________
Effect of return to work? ______________________
Workers' Compensation claim? ______________________
Previous job(s)? ______________ How long? ______________

Previous Treatment

1. Plant dispensary ______________________
2. Other physician ______________________
____
3. Self-treatment ______________________
____

Description of Work

____
____
____
____
Materials contacted ______________________
____
____
Other workers affected? Yes __________ No __________ No affected __________
How many workers on this job? ______________________
Methods of cleaning skin at work (and frequency) ______________________
____
Protective creams (names) ______________________
____
Protective clothing (incl. gloves) ______________________

Figure 10-4. A sample template for examination of patients with suspect occupational skin diseases.

Past History

Previous compensation claims? Yes _____ No _____ Explain _____

Previous skin diseases _____
Relation to occupation? Yes _____ No _____ Place of birth _____
Past health _____
Allergic history. Hay fever _____ Asthma _____ Eczema _____ Allergic to cosmetics, medications, creams, ointments, jewelry, drugs, perfumes? (circle which)
Describe _____
Family history of atopy or psoriasis? Yes _____ No _____ Second job _____

Hobbies

Contacts at Home

Housework _____ Full-time _____ Part-time _____
Married _____ Single _____ Widow _____ Divorced _____
Children _____ Yes _____ Number _____ Ages _____
Emotional factors _____

Physical Examination

General appearance _____

Description of disease _____

Other skin diseases _____

Diagnosis

Eczema	Yes _____	No _____	Different _____
Contact dermatitis	Entirely _____	Partially _____	No _____
Endogenous dermatitis	Atopic _____	Discoid _____	Seborrheic _____
	Hand _____	Foot _____	Asteatotic _____
	Face _____	Stasis _____	Unclassified _____

Pre–Patch Test Diagnosis

Sensitizers   Relevance
Irritants   Relevance
Occupational   Yes _____ No _____ Don't know _____

Special Tests

KOH _____ Fungal culture _____ Bacterial culture _____
Biopsy _____
Patch testing (results)   Sensitizers _____
                          Relevance _____
Occupational Yes _____ No _____ Clinical photographs? Yes _____ No _____
Treatment _____

Disability Yes _____ No _____ Occupational Yes _____ No _____
Remarks and Recommendations _____

Post–Patch Test Diagnosis

Sensitizers _____   Relevance _____
Irritants _____   Relevance _____
Occupational _____   Yes _____ No _____

Figure 10-4. (Continued)

Most states require the physician to file a *first report of occupational injury/illness* with the worker's compensation insurance carrier when he determines such illness/injury to be present (Figure 10-5). This report enables the insurance carrier and the employer to be formally notified of the worker's illness. It is essential information to enable the insurance carrier to provide benefits to the worker. Periodic supplemental reports are routinely required by insurance carriers in order to determine the worker's right to continued benefits.

The employer may be allowed to determine where the injured worker can seek medical attention. States will vary as to these rights. Physicians may have to be selected from a state-approved list, full control may be given to the employer, or the worker may have a waiting period (e.g., 30 days) prior to being allowed his choice of a health care provider.

When the patient's degree of impairment is evaluated by the physician, care should be taken to consider and comment only on the patient's degree of physical limitations. In contrast, disability must take into account all factors which may limit the patient's ability to work. Social factors such as level of education, alternative occupations available, and age to retirement are some of the nonmedical factors considered by insurance carriers and worker's compensation boards when attempting to quantitate disability. It is reasonable for the physician to comment on social factors that he strongly feels should be considered by disability evaluating boards.

The treating physician's aim should always be to return the worker to full employment without loss of wages. During the treatment period, a worker may be *temporarily totally disabled*. In this case, he would not be able to return to full or light duty. It is also the physician's responsibility to aid the patient in obtaining replacement salary benefits through the worker's compensation insurance carrier by keeping the adjuster fully informed. The healing period continues until either the worker is able to return to work or it is determined that his condition will no longer change with treatment (*permanent disability*).

Often workers' compensation insurance adjusters will ask at what point a worker becomes "permanent and stationary." This is the point at which a patient's condition is not expected to change significantly. One must remember that this is only an estimate. If a worker's previously stable dermatologic condition becomes unexpectedly worse, his case can always be reevaluated.

If a worker is determined by the insurance carrier or worker's compensation board to be permanently disabled, a professional disability evaluator is often utilized to determine what vocational rehabilitation is indicated. The physician's determination of medical impairment is pivotal in helping to determine appropriate alternative occupations.

A worker who is unable to work is considered permanently disabled and entitled to compensation. If a worker is only partially disabled and precluded from employment in a limited number of occupations, he is considered *permanently partially disabled*.

The Americans With Disabilities Act of 1990 asserts that the employer must make "reasonable accommodations" to allow prospective employees to perform job tasks. This act may have implications especially for physicians

STATE OF CALIFORNIA

DOCTOR'S FIRST REPORT OF OCCUPATIONAL INJURY OR ILLNESS

Within 5 days of your initial examination, for every occupational injury or illness, send this report to **insurer or employer (only if self-insured).** Failure to file a timely doctor's report may result in assessment of a civil penalty. **In the case of diagnosed or suspected pesticide poisoning,** send one copy of this report directly to the Division of Labor Statistics and Research, P.O. Box 603, San Francisco CA 94101; and notify your local health officer by telephone within 24 hours and by sending a copy of this report within seven days. For a supply of this form, please call (415) 557-1924.

1. **INSURER NAME AND ADDRESS**
2. **EMPLOYER NAME**
3. Address: No. and Street — City — Zip
4. Nature of business (e.g., food manufacturing, building construction, retailer of women's clothes)
5. **PATIENT NAME** (First name, middle initial, last name)
6. Sex ☐ Male ☐ Female
7. Date of Birth Mo. Day Yr.
8. Address: No. and Street — City — Zip
9. Telephone number ( )
10. Occupation (Specific job title)
11. Social Security Number - -
12. Injured at: No. and Street — City — County
13. Date and hour of injury or onset of illness Mo. Day Yr. Hour ______ a.m. ______ p.m.
14. Date last worked Mo. Day Yr.
15. Date and hour of first examination or treatment Mo. Day Yr. Hour ______ a.m. ______ p.m.
16. Have you (or your office) previously treated patient? ☐ Yes ☐ No

PLEASE DO NOT USE THIS COLUMN: Case No — Industry — County — Age — Hazard — Disease — Hospitalization — Occupation — Return Date/Code

Patient please complete this portion, if able to do so. Otherwise, doctor please complete immediately. Inability or failure of a patient to complete this portion shall not affect his/her rights to workers' compensation under the California Labor Code.

17. **DESCRIBE HOW THE ACCIDENT OR EXPOSURE HAPPENED** (Give specific object, machinery or chemical. Use reverse side if more space is required.)

18. **SUBJECTIVE COMPLAINTS** (Describe fully. Use reverse side if more space is required.)

19. **OBJECTIVE FINDINGS** (Use reverse side if more space is required.)
    A. Physical examination
    B. X-ray and laboratory results (State if none or pending.)

20. **DIAGNOSIS** (If occupational illness, specify etiologic agent and duration of exposure.) Chemical or toxic compounds involved? ☐ Yes ☐ No

21. Are your findings and diagnosis consistent with patient's account of injury or onset of illness? ☐ Yes ☐ No
    If "no", please explain.

22. Is there any other current condition that will impede or delay patient's recovery? ☐ Yes ☐ No
    If "yes", please explain.

23. **TREATMENT RENDERED** (Use reverse side if more space is required.)
    If further treatment required, specify treatment. Estimated duration

24. If hospitalized as inpatient, give hospital name and location. Date admitted Mo. Day Yr. Estimated stay

25. **WORK STATUS** Is patient able to perform usual work? ☐ Yes ☐ No
    If "no", patient can return to: Mo. Day Yr.
    Regular work ______
    Modified work ______ Specify restrictions ______

Doctor's Signature ______ Date ______ CA License Number ______
Doctor Name and Degree (Please Type) ______ IRS Number ______
Address ______ Telephone Number ( )

FORM 5021 (Rev. 3) 1989

Incomplete information or delay in submitting this report may cause delay in benefits to your patient.

Figure 10-5. When an occupational injury or illness is suspected, a physician's first report must be filed with the patient's workmans' compensation insurance carrier.

working with employed persons suffering from contact allergens and occupational skin disease.[9]

SUMMARY

The dermatologist should not be intimidated by the apparent complexity of practicing occupational dermatology or resist taking time from the office schedule to perform occasional workplace visits. Patients spend much of their time in the workplace environment and, not unexpectedly, often develop problems associated with occupational exposures. All working patients should be queried about such exposures as part of a complete medical and dermatologic evaluation.

REFERENCES

1. Mathias CG: Contact dermatitis and workers' compensation: Criteria for establishing occupational causation and aggravation. *J Am Acad Dermatol* 20:842–848, 1989.
2. US Department of Labor, Occupational Safety and Health Administration: *Report of the Advisory Committee on Cutaneous Hazards*. Washington, DC, US Government Printing Office, 1978.
3. Hogan D, Dannaker C, Maibach, H: Contact dermatitis: Prognosis, risk factors, and rehabilitation. *Semin Dermatol* 9:233–246, 1990.
4. Cohen SR: Sources of information for occupational dermatology. *Dermatol Clin*, 6:15–19, 1988.
5. American Conference of Governmental Industrial Hygienists: 1993–1994 threshold limit values for chemical substances and physical agents and biological exposure indices. American Conference of Governmental Industrial Hygienists, Cincinnati, 1993.
6. American Conference of Governmental Industrial Hygienists: Guide to occupational exposure values—1993. American Conference of Governmental Industrial Hygienists, Cincinnati, 1993.
7. LaDou J (ed): *Occupational Medicine*. Englewood Cliffs, NJ, Prentice-Hall, 1990.
8. Adams R: *Occupational Skin Disease*, ed 2. WB Saunders, Philadelphia, 1990.
9. Nethercott JR: The Americans With Disabilities Act of 1990. *Am J Contact Dermatitis* 4:185–186, 1993.

11

Dealing with Workers' Compensation Boards

Douglas A. Swanson

The objectives of most workers' compensation systems are:

1. To provide sure and prompt medical care and reasonable replacement income to injured workers, *regardless* of fault.
2. To provide a relatively rapid administrative system to deliver medical care and compensation.
3. To restore the injured worker, physically and economically, to a self-sufficient status.

With these objectives in mind, it is the purpose of this chapter to provide the medical dermatologist with a brief overview of workers' compensation systems and a framework for writing reports that will be utilized by insurance companies, workers' compensation lawyers, and workers' compensation judges.

There are two primary points to keep in mind when providing reports on behalf of an injured worker.

First, all workers' compensation systems are *no-fault*. This simply means that the injured worker is to be compensated for his or her injury without regard to whose fault it is, the employer's or the employee's. Therefore, if the worker is somehow negligent in exposing the body to an offending substance, such negligence should not defeat the claim. The only test is whether the injury is work related. Contrast this situation to an auto accident case in which a person cannot recover for injuries unless he or she proves that another person is at fault.

Second, the worker has the *burden of proving* that the injury is work related. The worker must produce medical evidence connecting the work exposure with the injury. In the workers' compensation setting, such medical evidence is almost always produced by the treating doctor, either by generating a report or by giving a deposition. If the claim has been denied by the insurance company and the treating doctor is unwilling or unable to provide such a report or deposition, the injured worker will not be able to prove that he or she has a work-related problem.

With these two principles in mind, let's consider the confluence of medical and legal terminology found in almost all workers' compensation systems.

WORKERS' COMPENSATION TERMS[1]

Aggravation.
1. Recurrence or worsening of a once-stationary compensable condition without intervening accident or disease;
2. As a result of work activity or exposure:
   a. manifestation of a latent, underlying condition which was previously asymptomatic; or,
   b. worsening of a manifest preexisting condition.

Compensability. Means the condition is covered under the workers' compensation law as an injury or disease which arose out of and in the course of employment. Relates to causation question.

Disabling Claim. Condition is considered disabling if:
1. Worker is required to remain off work during the healing period (temporary disability); or
2. If permanent disability (either partial or total) or death results.

Disability. An administrative or judicial evaluation of the patient's ability to perform the activities of daily living and/or work as affected by permanent medical impairment and by social factors such as age, sex, education, training, and work experience. Refers to an incapacity, because of the injury or disease, to earn the wage previously earned by the worker, or to perform past work. May also refer to loss or impairment of physical or mental function.

Impairment. Purely medical evaluation of loss or abnormality of psychological, physiological, or anatomical structure or function, including a specifically acquired altered immunological capacity to react, which does not remit nor is likely to remit after a period of reasonable medical treatment and rehabilitation.

Medically Stationary. No further material improvement would reasonably be

	expected from further medical treatment or the passage of time.
Occupational Disease.	Disease or infection which arises out of and in the course of employment due to continued or repeated exposure to workplace hazards (e.g., dermatitis, asbestosis).
Occupational Injury.	Injury arising out of and in the course of employment resulting from the unexpected results of exertion and strain or trauma of violent or external means (e.g., fracture, laceration).
Permanency.	May refer to situation in which: 1. Signs of skin disease will continue to be present; or 2. Recurrence is inevitable with reexposure to allergens or irritants, making avoidance of offending substances essential.
Reasonable Medical Probability.	Legal standard which must be satisfied for condition to be considered compensable. Means the likelihood that a given condition or illness was caused by the particular employment is greater than 50 percent. (Possibility implies a less than 50% likelihood that the condition was caused by employment.)
Scheduled Injury.	Definition used in connection with disability ratings. Refers to injuries to body parts or organs specifically enumerated in statutory schedules (e.g., hands, arms, legs, feet, eyes, ears). Payments are fixed for loss of specified member or loss of function equal to partial loss regardless of effect on earning capacity.
Sensitization.	1. Medical definition: allergy. 2. Medico-legal definition: Refers to a worker's skin having become fragile or vulnerable to a specific substance or group of substances, not necessarily because of an allergic reaction, but which nonetheless requires avoidance of that substance.
Systemic.	1. Medical definition: Involvement of organ systems, as heart, lungs, etc. 2. Medico-legal definition: Entire skin surface is susceptible to reaction if exposed to the offending substance. Allergic contact dermatitis is an example of systemic skin disease; irritant dermatitis is not.
Unmasking.	In the context of skin disease, refers to situation in which an atopic person, whose condition was previously latent, develops dermatitis as a result of the work environment which thereafter may become a persistent problem. (See Aggravation 2[a].)
Unscheduled Injury.	Definition used in connection with disability ratings. Injuries or diseases affecting body parts not enumer-

ated in the statutory schedules are considered unscheduled (e.g., back injuries, psychiatric problems). Disability is evaluated upon impairment of the whole person and requires evaluation of loss of earning capacity as affected by the physical impairment and social factors, including age, sex, education, training, and work experience.

CAUSATION QUESTIONS

The most important report a doctor provides addresses the question of whether or not the work exposure caused, at least in part, the dermatitic injury. Without such a report, the worker simply will not have a workers' compensation claim. A good compensability report must include the following:

1. The patient's occupational history. This means that you must be aware of the nature of the patient's job and understand what chemicals or other offending substances the patient was exposed to.
2. The relevant medical history. This should include the history of any prior dermatologic conditions, allergies, or atopy; the date of the first contact with the irritants or allergens; and a review of the present condition. It's important to note whether or not the patient has suffered any previous eruptions, in either the same or different work, and if the patient has improved with withdrawal from work and has suffered recurrence with occupational exposure.
3. Note off-the-job exposures or allergens and compare them to on-the-job exposures or allergens.
4. Discuss other cases with which you may be familiar or literature with which you may be familiar relating to the patient's problem.
5. Describe the patch tests applied and the results. Attach copies of the test results.
6. Diagnosis. Clearly state your diagnosis. You can indicate here whether this is work related and if the condition is irritant or allergic.
7. Conclusion. State your opinion as to whether or not this condition is work related. If you believe the condition is work related, explain your reasoning. If there are off-the-job exposures to offending substances, compare the degree and intensity of on-the-job versus off-the-job exposures. Discuss the relationship between preexisting skin conditions and the present condition, if appropriate. Explain if the present industrial exposure worsened, accelerated, aggravated, or unmasked the condition.
8. Indicate whether the claim is disabling. Indicate whether or not the patient should remain away from work during the recovery or, if appropriate, indicate that the patient can work but cannot work near certain

substances. This is generally referred to as *light duty* work or *restricted work*.

9. Indicate the long-term prognosis. Is this an allergic reaction such that the patient must avoid all contact with the substance in the future? Or is it an acute irritant reaction that should subside without permanency?

10. Is the worker *medically stationary* or *stable* (i.e., has the worker achieved *maximum medical improvement*?)? In workers' compensation, those phrases generally mean the same thing, and the phrase you use will generally depend on your state laws. The phrases basically mean that no further medical improvement can be expected with either the passage of time or further medical treatment. Once the worker is medically stationary, permanent impairment can be rated.

11. Permanent impairment. You must address the degree of permanent impairment, if appropriate. It is at this stage that the distinction between impairment and disability comes into play (see "Workers' Compensation Terms"). It is important to keep in mind that *impairment* is a medical term and *disability* is a social/vocational term. (For example, a 60-year-old concrete finisher may develop a mild to moderate skin impairment but may be totally disabled because of his particular social/vocational factors of no formal education and having performed only this work throughout his life. However, a 60-year-old architect may have developed the same sensitivity and may also have a mild to moderate skin impairment, but may not suffer any disability because of his better education and ability to work in a setting which can be more controlled.)

In Section 11 of the report, it is important to discuss whether or not the dermatitis is allergic (systemic) or irritant (affecting only that part of the body that comes into contact with the offending substance).

Most American workers' compensation systems recognize, on one level or another, the American Medical Association's *Guides to the Evaluation of Permanent Impairment*.[4] The *Guides* contain the criteria for evaluating permanent impairment of the skin and are accompanied by numerous examples.

In Section 11 of the report, it is important to note how the impairment affects the patient's work life. You should indicate whether or not the worker can return to his or her employment at all or in a restricted work capacity. If there are reasonable modifications the employer can make to accommodate the worker, suggestions from the treating physician are generally appropriate.

SAMPLE LETTERS[2]

The following example is taken from a chart note that does an excellent job of relating the patient's allergic contact dermatitis to his work as a photography professor. Because the case was contested by the insurance company, the patient's attorney felt it necessary to follow up on the chart note and asked the doctor a series of specific questions, to which he responded.

In the chart note, see that the doctor paid particular attention to the question of the preexisting atopic condition and how it related to the developing allergic contact dermatitis.

> The patient came to ask for help in determining what component of his long-time dermatitis was allergic contact dermatitis compared to his life-long atopic dermatitis. He clearly has had atopic dermatitis from infancy.
>
> He recalls that he had waxing and waning of his dermatitis and that it was better for the first few months when he was first married and moved here, but he always noted more irritation when exposed to photo-related chemicals. His testing had also shown allergy to cats, acacia trees, peanuts and many other allergens—
>
> The reactions that he noticed to chemicals were relatively briefer in the past, but beginning 10 years ago, it seemed to take him longer to get over the insults. He notes that the onset was also sooner in the past, possibly within one to eight hours, whereas the onset now is 12 to 24 hours. This change in onset also began about 10 years ago and it was at that time that he began cutting down on his "own creative work" and he tapered off dark room work gradually until about five years ago when he consciously stopped the serious work. He was doing only occasional prints and that postponed dealing with his problem. Thus, he feels a qualitative change began in his dermatitis approximately 10 years ago and increased even more dramatically five years ago.
>
> He also has made observations about the quantitative aspects of his previous work exposures. Prior to his working at City College and State University, his photographic developing was primarily in the gallon-sized range and required relatively little contact with the skin. When he began teaching, the magnitude increased five-fold; i.e., five gallons exposure per week and he also began working with dichromate and gum arabic mixtures which involved considerable contact with the hands and close exposure when viewing and applying these materials. The number of prints also increased considerably to perhaps at times 150 prints per day from the students versus eight prints on occasion at home when he would be printing. Also, with the teaching, he had to mix the chemicals himself and do all of the dark room work himself, including painting tables and cabinets with epoxy paint on the dark room sinks, etc. His work at the universities also expanded from 60 students originally to 175 students per quarter.
>
> I explained to Mr. Smith that he has had the unusual condition of having two types of allergic hypersensitivity. He probably was born with atopic dermatitis which is sometimes referred to as an "intrinsic" dermatitis and then at some point later he developed the extrinsic allergic contact dermatitis to photo developers, chromate and possibly other materials as well. It appears that he had typical atopic dermatitis and, from the multiple positive skin tests, was extremely atopic. Probably his skin was sensitive to any number of irritants through the years as well. He occasionally noted this irritation throughout the time that he was working at City College and State University. I would estimate this was most likely an irritative phenomenon rather than an overt allergy because of the rapid onset and the very rare instances of immediate hypersensitivity to chemicals such as CD3, chromates, etc. Through the years of his work exposure, he always noted a clear temporal association with the days of the week when he was in class. Probably the critical change point occurred approximately 10 years ago when

he began developing lesions that, rather than being brief, became much more lasting, consistent with allergic contact dermatitis.

Since his last appointment, I received a report of a consultation by Dr. Brown on February 8, 1991. Dr. Brown elicited the history that the patient first noted having allergic problems following exposure to photography chemicals in the 1960's and consisting of palmar vesicles with extension of the rash to the elbows and also extension on to the neck and face and occasionally into axillae chest and legs. A problem seems to be the interpretation of the term "allergic problems." It seems more likely that this was a flare of his atopic dermatitis, possibly exacerbated by chemical exposure but by no means evidence of allergic contact dermatitis, especially with the history of problems on the palms rather than on the dorsal surfaces. Improvement during vacation times is also no sure proof of allergic contact dermatitis, since atopic dermatitis often improves during vacations and removal from stress. Only in the past two to three years has the patient actually noted definitive problems with welting when chemicals were spilled on the arms, according to an evaluation by Dr. Brown. Part of the problem with Dr. Brown's evaluation is that he noted positive reactions to potassium dichromate and epoxy but did not see the strongly positive responses to the developers that we elicited at the time of patch testing. There is also confusion as to the current diagnosis which he states is "contact dermatitis," which is congenital and not related to Mr. Smith's occupation. There is a problem here with definition of terms, and it is unclear whether he means irritant contact dermatitis or allergic contact dermatitis. Regardless, contact dermatitis is not congenital. In the next response as to etiology of the diagnosis, he states that the cause is the atopic dermatitis which is a congenital condition. There is also considerable question about his response to the third question, stating that exposure to potential vapors are not consistent with development of contact dermatitis and this simply is not true. Certainly, his overall condition has improved markedly since the patient has been avoiding these chemicals and at the present time he shows minimal evidence of any dermatitis. I certainly agree with Dr. Brown's suggestion that the atopic dermatitis can limit the patient's ability to work in the dark room directly with photographic chemicals due to irritation, but the question of allergic aggravation again is poorly defined. Dr. Brown was not aware of the fact that the patient had allergic contact dermatitis. It appears that he is referring to immediate-type airborne allergies often associated with dermatitis but probably irrelevant in the dark room.

In the follow-up letter, some of the questions might seem redundant. Since a workers' compensation judge was to review the medical record in order to determine whether or not the condition was work related, the patient's attorney felt that the condition and its cause needed to be clearly stated. It was also important to show that the reports of the doctors retained by the insurance company were considered and, if appropriate, refuted:

Dear Mr. Attorney:

I am responding to your specific questions regarding the diagnosis of Mr. Smith's skin condition:

1. Please clarify that allergic contact dermatitis is a distinct entity from atopic dermatitis.

    Definitely allergic contact dermatitis is a distinct entity. It is a specific immunologic reaction to a chemical applied to the skin, whereas atopic

dermatitis is a non-specific hyperreactivity to all manner of exacerbants, including infection, emotional stress, irritants and allergens.
2. Please indicate that the allergic contact dermatitis has actually been caused by his work-related exposures and is therefore a completely work-related condition. Please indicate that you have reviewed the file, you have reviewed Dr. Milton's and Dr. Butter's reports, and it continues to be your strong opinion that Mr. Smith's allergic contact dermatitis was caused by his work exposures.
    i. The patient has allergic contact dermatitis, documented by patch testing, to chemicals that are present in his work environment.
    ii. His dermatitis continued whenever he was exposed to his work chemicals.
    iii. The dermatitis remitted when he avoided contact with those chemicals. This is definitive evidence for work-related allergic contact dermatitis.

    I have reviewed the consultations by Drs. Milton and Butters. Dr. Butters apparently was not aware of the patch testing information showing allergic contact dermatitis. Dr. Milton recognized the diagnosis of allergic contact dermatitis and atopic dermatitis. Both consultants demonstrated some ambiguity in distinguishing between allergic contact dermatitis and atopic dermatitis. Atopic dermatitis is a condition that usually comes on early in life and, from the patient's history, this form of dermatitis was clearly active during his early years. This is a constitutional condition and the predisposed individual is subject to recurrent exacerbations of atopic dermatitis for many years, sometimes throughout life. Thus, Mr. Smith had both conditions and that is quite unusual. The fact that Mr. Smith's dermatitis remitted when he began avoiding the chemicals that caused his allergic contact dermatitis indicates that the previous, constitutional atopic dermatitis is not presently active.
3. My understanding is that you have treated Mr. Smith for approximately one year now, and he essentially has no atopic dermatitis.

    See above. I have treated Mr. Smith since February 4, 1992. I cannot say that he has no atopic dermatitis, since it is a lifelong constitutional trait, but he apparently has no *active* atopic dermatitis at the present time (I have not seen the patient since June 2, 1992).
4. Was Mr. Smith taking steroids to control his work-related allergic contact dermatitis?

    The best treatment of work-related allergic contact dermatitis is avoidance of the specific allergenic chemicals. Since the diagnosis of allergic contact dermatitis had not been made at the time he was treated with steroids, that therapy was apparently directed at a presumptive diagnosis of atopic dermatitis. In retrospect, Mr. Smith had allergic contact dermatitis and the steroids were being given to control that dermatitis.
5. After treating Mr. Smith for a year, please explain how your treatment and his response to that treatment confirm your diagnosis. In other words, has Mr. Smith improved once he was restricted from working around chemicals?

    See above (answer to #2). Yes, Mr. Smith has improved after restricting his contact with chemicals to which he has contact allergy.

If you have other questions or need clarifications of the above answers, please feel free to call on me.

SAMPLE LETTERS

The following example is from a slightly different perspective. The doctor who authored the report was asked to provide a consulting opinion to the state insurance fund. From the report, it can be seen that the examining doctor reviewed the treating doctor's records and noted the treating doctor's patch testing. In her report, the consulting doctor indicates that she patch-tested the patient again, and then clearly points out that the chromatic exposure at work was the cause of this patient's allergic contact dermatitis.

Dear Ms. Claims Adjuster:

I was happy to see the patient on June 30, and July 2, 1994. You know that he first injured his right thumb in October of 1992 while working as a cement finisher. He had worked as a cement finisher since September, 1991. The original injury "never healed" and developed into an extensive hand eczema with patches of eczema occurring elsewhere on his body as well. It became such a severe problem that he finally stopped working as a cement finisher on December 28, 1993, and he has not worked since that day. His back was involved in July, 1993, after he was patch tested and it then cleared for six months. The involvement of his back returned approximately a week ago.

During this period of time, the patient has been cared for by Dr. Jones, who has documented his chromate sensitivity and has treated him with a variety of topical and systemic corticosteroids. Dr. Jones has frequently worked with your office in an effort to secure retraining for the patient in a chrome-free environment.

The patient has a father with asthma and hay fever but no eczema. He himself has never had any asthma or hay fever, nor did he have eczema as a child, according to a conversation he had with his mother while he was under my care.

On the 30th of June, the patient had a patchy, nummular, eczematous dermatitis in several spots on his hands. His back was involved diffusely with plaques of a serpiginous, scaling, eczematous looking eruption which was KOH negative on several tries. His feet and legs, scalp and face were all clear.

I was certainly satisfied with Dr. Jones's records and presentation as an example of a chromate contact dermatitis. I did, however, repatch him to nickel, chrome and cobalt in an effort to document this, as you evidently were seeking a second opinion. I saw the patient a second time on July 2nd and Dr. Jones has seen him on July 1st. He had an exquisitely positive chromate patch which I have documented with photographs and will include one of them with this letter, but it is possible that his cobalt will come up. He is instructed to return on July 7th if either of these two patch tests are positive, and I will so inform you. Dr. Jones biopsied his back on the first of July to rule out the unlikely possibility that he was developing psoriasis as well as eczema, and we will include a copy of that biopsy report for your information as well. The real issue at stake here, however, is what to do with the patient's chromate contact dermatitis. Men who work in the cement business who become sensitive to chromate have one devil of a time ridding themselves of this problem. Typically, chromate contact dermatitis lasts far longer than exposure to chromate. By far longer I mean years. It is not unusual for these men to develop plaques of eczema on many parts of their body where chrome never touches them. This seems to be one of those allergic contact dermatitis problems that in a way is "systemic." Despite the most conscientious efforts of these people to avoid chrome in their work and their personal environments, they do indeed tend to continue to have difficulties despite chrome avoidance. It should be pointed out that chrome can be found in a great number of places in our environment and for your information as well, I will include the sort of information sheet that we give to our chrome sensitive patients. This sheet does not mean that chrome is definitely found in all of these areas, but that it may be.

In summary then, the patient is likely to have contact dermatitis on his hands and here and there on his body for many years to come, no matter what line of work he engages in. This does not mean, however, that he cannot work. Indeed, if he works in as chrome-free an environment as one can find and if he will avoid very wet work, he is likely to do as well as can be expected. He may, from time to time, have acute flare-ups of his eczema, but this can be treated with systemic and topical corticosteroids and he can continue to work. Some sort of office work, warehouse work, maintenance work, or security work would be ideal. Surely, the industrial hygienist employed by the workman's compensation people could assist in this regard.

The final example involves another request for consultation by the state insurance fund. Note that the physician initially indicates that additional information is needed. This is important to ensure that the physician's report is complete and that she arrived at her opinion with full knowledge of the medical history.

Note further that the doctor indicated that there was "probably" a causal relationship. Remember that *reasonable medical probability* is the legal standard that must be satisfied. *Possible* or *possibilities* are generally not considered legally significant. *Probable* simply means "more likely than not," a 51% chance or more. Scientific certainty is not required in the legal arena.

Dear Mr. Claims Adjuster:
I have reviewed the information you provided me concerning Mr. Turner. Several important pieces of information are absent from that report:
1. Is Mr. Turner an atopic, i.e., does he or do members of his family have asthma, hay fever or eczema in their present or past medical histories?
2. Does Mr. Turner have varicose veins in either his right or left leg?
3. Had he ever had any leg edema or leg eczema before his 6/20/92 injury?
4. Has the possibility of the use of topical agents (other than steroids or Tinactin) on his legs after the 6/20/92 injury been carefully excluded?

If the answers to my questions 1 through 3 are "No" and to question 4 is "Yes," then I would answer the question you put to me as follows:

Yes, I would say there is probably a direct causal relationship between Mr. Turner's 6/20/92 injury and his present "eczema condition." The lateral malleoli are particularly prone to develop stasis dermatitis, especially in the setting of deep tissue injury and longstanding peripheral edema of the sort described in your report. Once this condition begins, it tends to be chronic, to be associated with further local injury, to frequently develop "flare ups" which we seldom explain very well, to become secondarily infected and often sensitized and, finally, to become associated with extensive patches of eczema on the body (so-called auto-eczematization or "id" reactions). Again, we don't explain this situation very well, but it is a definite and reproducible clinical experience. If Mr. Turner had no prior eczema or a history of it, no varicosities, no peripheral edema, then his crushing leg injury on 6/20/92 could have permanently altered the deep tissues in his left leg under the supramalleolar skin in such a way that he may have trouble with stasis dermatitis and even stasis ulcers there for the rest of his life.

It is very unlikely that an underlying medical problem is causing this difficulty, unless, of course, Mr. Turner is a roaring atopic, and even then his atopy would probably be only partially responsible.

From my above comments you can tell that the precise etiology of stasis dermatitis is not perfectly understood. However, tissue injury with consequent edema, vascular compromise and secondary infection are all factors which participate in the development of this chronic problem.

Leg elevation, lubrication, support such as an ace wrap, topical steroids for eczema, and systemic antibiotics for infections should all assist Mr. Turner in maintaining a leg that he can work on easily, but he is likely to have medical problems related to this difficulty for many years to come.

I do hope my comments are helpful. Don't hesitate to contact me further.

CONCLUSION

Letters discussing occupational skin disease obviously vary greatly among authors and depending on whether the report is rendered for a patient or as a consulting exam. However, addressing most, if not all, of the points raised here will go a long way toward addressing questions that insurers, attorneys, and judges will have concerning occupationally related skin disease. Next to providing treatment for your patient, producing a thorough, well-written report detailing the work-related problem may be the most important service you can give.

REFERENCES

1. This chapter is based on and quotes extensively from Goldstein A: Writing report letters for patients with skin disease resulting from on-the-job exposures, *Dermatologic Clinics* 2:631–641, 1984. The "Workers' Compensation Terms" and the section "Causation Questions" are from this article.
2. The medical reports used as examples were authored by Dr. Jon Hanifin and Dr. Francis Storrs, both professors of dermatology at Oregon Health Science University in Portland, Oregon.

BIBLIOGRAPHY

1. Adams RM: High risk dermatoses. *J Occup Med* 23:829–834, 1981.
2. Adams RM: The diagnosis of occupational skin disease. In Maibach HI, Gellin GA (eds): *Occupational and Industrial Dermatology*. Chicago, Year Book Medical, 1982, p 2.

3. American Medical Association: *Guides to the Evaluation of Permanent Impairment,* ed 2. Chicago, American Medical Association, 1988, p 2.
4. Larson A: *The Law of Workmen's Compensation.* New York, Matthew Bender, 1982–1983, section 1, 6, 12, 29, 37, 41, 57, 58, 83 and Appendix B, Tables 2, 2A, 6, 13, and 15.
5. Whitmore CW, Adams RM: Medicolegal aspects. In Adams RM: *Occupational Skin Disease.* San Francisco. Grune & Stratton, 1983, pp 179–188.

Appendix 1

North American Contact Dermatitis Group Standard Allergens

Benzocaine	5%	Methylchloroisothiazolinone/ methylisothiazolinone	100 ppm
Mercaptobenzothiazole	1%	Paraben mix	12%
Colophony (rosin)	20%	Methyldibromoglutaronitrile Phenoxyethanol	1%
P-Phenylenediamine	1%	Fragrance mix	8%
Imidazolidinyl urea	2%	Glutaraldehyde	2%
Cinnamic aldehyde	1%	2-Bromo-nitropropane-1, 3 diol	0.5%
Lanolin alcohol	30%	Sesquiterpene lactone mix	1%
Carba mix	3%	Thimerosal (merthiolate, thiomersal)	0.1%
Neomycin sulfate	20%	Propylene glycol (aqueous)	10%
Thiuram mix	1%	PCMX (4-Chloro-3, xylenol)	1%
Formaldehyde (aqueous)	1%	Ethyleneurea melamine formaldehyde	5%
Ethylenediamine dihydrochloride	1%	Phenoxyethanol	1%
Epoxy resin	1%	BHA (Butylated hydroxyanisole)	2%
Quaternium-15	2%	BHT (Butylated hydroxytoluene)	2%
P-tert-Butylphenol formaldehyde resin	1%	Ethyl acrylate	0.1%
Mercapto mix	1%	Glyceryl thioglycolate	1%
Black rubber mix	0.6%	Toluenesulfonamide formaldehyde resin	10%
Potassium dichromate	0.25%	Methyl methacrylate	2%
Balsam of Peru	25%	Cobalt chloride	1%
Nickel sulfate	2.5%	Tixocortol-21-pivalate	1%
Diazolidinyl urea	1%		
DMDM hydantoin	1%		
Bacitracin	20%		
Mixed dialkyl thiourea	1%		

PATCH TEST READING MORPHOLOGY CODES

Weak (non-vesicular) reaction erythema, infiltration, possibly papules (+)
Strong (edematous or vesicular) reaction (+ +)
Extreme (spreading, bullous, ulcerative) reaction (+ + +)

Macular erythema only (doubtful)
Irritant morphology (IR)
Negative reaction (−)
Not tested
Not done (for second reading)

True Test*

Allergen	Labelled amount micrograms/cm²
1. Nickel sulphate	200
2. Wool alcohols	1000
3. Neomycin sulphate	200
4. Potassium dichromate	25
5. Caine mix	700
6. Fragrance mix	450
7. Colophony	1500
8. Epoxy resin	50
9. Quinoline mix	200
10. Balsam of Peru	800
11. Ethylenediamine dihydrochloride	50
12. Cobalt chloride	20
13. *p-tert* Butylphenol formaldehyde resin	40
14. Paraben mix	1000
15. Carba mix	250
16. Black rubber mix	75
17. Cl+Me-Isothiazolinone (Kathon CG)	4
18. Quaternium-15	100
19. Mercaptobenzothiazole	75
20. *P*-Phenylenediamine	90
21. Formaldehyde	180
22. Mercapto mix	75
23. Thiomersal	8
24. Thiuram mix	25

Manufactured by:
Pharmacia AS
Hillerød, Denmark

*Thin-layer Rapid Use Epicutaneous Test. Currently available in Europe. Awaiting FDA approval, American version to be marketed by Glaxo Dermatology.

APPENDIX 1

Commercial Patch Test Trays Available from Chemotechnique and Hermal/Trolab

CHEMOTECHNIQUE

Medicament Series

Chloramphenicol	5.0
Kanamycin sulfate	10.0
Quinine sulfate	1.0
Sulfanilamide	5.0
Gentamicin sulfate	20.0
Nitrofurazone	1.0
Bacitracin	5.0
Polymyxin B sulfate	5.0
Caine mix III	10.0
Miconazole	1.0
Econazole nitrate	1.0
Caine mix IV	10.0

Corticosteroid Series

Budesonide	0.1
Betamethasone-17-valerate	1.0
Triamcinolone acetonide	1.0
Tixocortol-21-pivalate	1.0
Alclomethasone-17,21-dipropionate	1.0
Clobetasol-17-propionate	1.0

HERMAL/TROLAB

Medicaments

Benzoyl Peroxide	1
Resorcinol	2
Monobenzone (Hydroquinone Monobenzylether)	1
Propolis	10
Tylosin Tartrate	5
Phenyl Salicylate	1
Halquinol	1
Thiamine Hydrochloride (Vit. B1)	10
Pyridoxine Hydrochloride (Vit. B6)	10
Clioquinol (Chinoform)	5
Chlorquinaldol	5
Piperazine	1
Arrica Tincture	20
Bacitracin	20
Chloramphenicol	5
Gentamycin Sulphate	20
Nitrofurazone	1
Propantheline Bromide	5
Quinine Sulphate	1
Quinoline Yellow	0.1
Sulfanilamide	5

Local Anaesthetics

Procaine Hydrochloride	1
Cinchocaine Hydrochloride (Cincaine)	5
Tetracaine Hydrochloride (Amethocaine)	1
Lidocaine Hydrochloride	15

CHEMOTECHNIQUE

Corticosteroid Series (cont'd)

Dexamethasone-21-phosphate disodium salt	1.0
Hydrocortisone-17-butyrate	1.0

Hairdressing Series

4-Phenylenediamine base	1.0
2,5-Diaminotoluene sulfate	1.0
2-Nitro-4-phenylenediamine	1.0
Ammonium thioglycolate	2.5
Ammonium persulfate	2.5
Formaldehyde	1.0
Nickel sulfate	5.0
Cobalt chloride	1.0
Resorcinol	1.0
3-Aminophenol	1.0
4-Aminophenol	1.0
Hydrogen peroxide	3.0
Hydroquinone	1.0
Balsam Peru	25.0
Chloroacetamide	0.2
Glyceryl monothioglycolate (GMTG)	1.0
Cocamidopropylbetaine	1.0
Cl+Me-isothiazolinone (Kathon CG, 200 ppm)	1.34
2-Bromo-2-nitropropane-1,3-diol (Bronopol)	0.25
Captan	0.5
4-Chloro-3-cresol (PCMC)	1.0
4-Chloro-3-xylenol (PCMX)	0.5
Imidazolidinyl urea (Germall 115)	2.0
Quaternium 15 (Dowicil 200)	1.0
Zinc pyrithione (Zinc omadine)	1.0
Diazolidinylurea (Germall II)	2.0

Cosmetic Series

Isopropyl myristate	20.0
Amerchol L 101	100
Triethanolamine	2.0
Polyoxyethylenesorbitan oleate (Tween 80)	5.0

HERMAL/TROLAB

Hairdressing

o-Nitro-p-phenylenediamine	1
Resorcinol	2
p-Toluenediamine Sulphate	1
Glyceryl Monothioglycolate	1
Ammonium Thioglycolate	2.5
Ammonium Persulphate	2.5
p-Aminodiphenylamine Hydrochloride	0.25
Pyrogallol	1

Antimicrobials, Preservatives

Chlorocresol (PCMC)	1
Chloroxylenol (PCMX)	1
Bronopol	0.5
Imidazolidinyl Urea (Germall 115)	2

CHEMOTECHNIQUE

Cosmetic Series (cont'd)

Sorbitan monooleate (Span 80)	5.0
2-tert-Butyl-4-methoxyphenol (BHA)	2.0
2, 6-Ditert-Butyl-4-cresol (BHT)	2.0
Octyl gallate	0.25
Triclosan (Irgasan DP 300)	2.0
Sorbic Acid	2.0
4-Chloro-3-cresol (PCMC)	1.0
4-Chloro-3-xylenol (PCMX)	0.5
Thimerosal (Merthiolate)	0.1
Imidazolidinylurea (Germall 115)	2.0
Hexamethylenetetramine (Hexamin)	2.0
Chlorhexidine digluconate	0.5
Parabens	12.0
Phenylmercuric acetate	0.01
Chloroacetamide	0.2
Hexahydro-1,3,5-tris(hydroxyethyl) triazine (Grotan BK)	1.0
Clioquinol (5-chloro-7-iodo-quinolinol)	5.0
Ethylenediamine dihydrochloride	1.0
Abitol	10.0
Phenyl salicylate (Salol)	1.0
2-Hydroxy-4-methoxybenzophenone	2.0
Sorbitan sesquioleate (Arlacel 83)	20.0
Propylene glycol	5.0
Stearyl alcohol	30.0
Cetyl alcohol	5.0
Benzyl salicylate	2.0
2-Bromo-2-nitropropane-1,3-diol (Bronopol)	0.25
Sodium-2-pyridinethiol-1-oxide (Sodiumomadine)	0.1
Cocamidopropyl betaine	1.0
Benzyl alcohol	1.0
Cl + Me-isothiazolinone (Kathon CG, 200 ppm)	1.34
tert-Butylhydroquinone	1.0
2 (2-Hydroxy-5-methylphenyl) benzotriazol (Tinuvin P)	1.0
Propyl gallate	1.0

HERMAL/TROLAB

Antimicrobials, Preservatives (cont'd)

Butyl Hydroxytoluene (BHT)	2
Butyl Hydroxyanisole (BHA)	2
Phenylmercuric Acetate (in water)	0.01
Sorbic Acid	2
Chlorhexidine Digluconate (in water)	0.5
Chloramine T (in water)	0.5
Chloracetamide	0.2
Glutaraldehyde	1
1,3,5-Tris(2-hydroxyethyl)-hexahydrotriazine	1
2-Chloro-N-hydroxy Methylacetamide	0.2
Thiomersal	0.1
Phenylmercuric Nitrate (in water)	0.01
Clioquinol (Chinoform)	5
Chlorquinaldol	5
Methyl Parahydroxybenzoate	3
Ethyl Parahydroxybenzoate	3
Propyl Parahydroxybenzoate	3
Butyl Parahydroxybenzoate	3
Benzyl Parahydroxybenzoate	3
Benzalkonium Chloride (in water)	0.1
Hexyl Resorcinol	0.25
Triclosan	2
Benzotriazole	1

Vehicles, Emulsifiers

Eucerin®	100
Trolamine (Triethanolamine)	2.5
Propylene glycol	2
Sorbitan Sesquioleate	20
Cetyl stearyl alcohol	20
Amerchol® L 101	50
Polyoxyethylene Sorbitan Monopalmitate	10
Polyoxyethylene Sorbitan Monooleate	10

CHEMOTECHNIQUE

Cosmetic Series (cont'd)

Dodecyl gallate	0.25
Quaternium 15 (Dowicil 200)	1.0
2-Phenoxyethanol	1.0
Diazolidinylurea (Germall II)	2.0
Euxyl K 400	0.5
DMDM Hydantoin	2.0

Sunscreen Series

4-tert. Butyl-4'-methoxy-dibenzoylmethane (Parsol® 1789)	2.0
4-Aminobenzoic acid (PABA)	5.0
4-Isopropyl-dibenzoylmethane (Eusolex® 8020)	2.0
3-(4-Methylbenzyliden)camphor (Eusolex® 6300)	2.0
2-Ethylhexyl-4-dimethylaminobenzoate (Eusolex® 6007, Escalol 507, Octyl Dimethyl-PABA)	2.0
2-Hydroxy-4-methoxybenzophenone (Eusolex® 4360, Escalol® 567, Oxybenzone)	2.0
2-Ethylhexyl-4-methoxycinnamate (Parsol® MCX, Escalol® 557)	2.0
2-Hydroxy-methoxymethylbenzophenone (Mexenone)	2.0
2-Phenylbenzimidazol-5-sulfonic acid (Eusolex® 232, Novantisol)	2.0
2-Hydroxy-4-methoxybenzophenon-5-sulfonic acid (Sulisobenzone, Uvinyl MS-40, Benzophenone 4)	5.0

Fragrance Series

Cinnamic aldehyde	1.0
Cinnamic alcohol	2.0

HERMAL/TROLAB

Sunscreen Agents

1-(4-Isopropylphenyl)-3-Phenyl-1, 3-Propanedione (Eusolex® 8020)	2
4-tert-Butyl-4'-Methoxy-Dibenzoylmethane (Parsol® 1789)	2
p-Aminobenzoic Acid	2
2-Ethylhexyl-p-Dimethylaminobenzoate (Escalol® 507)	2
2-Ethylhexyl-p-Methoxycinnamate (Parsol® MCX)	2
2-Ethoxyethyl-p-Methoxycinnamate (Giv Tan® F)	2
3-(4-Methylbenzylidene)-Camphor (Eusolex® 6300)	2
Oxybenzone (Eusolex® 4360)	2

Perfumes, Flavors

Benzyl Salicylate	1
Clove Oil	2

CHEMOTECHNIQUE

Fragrance Series (cont'd)

Amylcinnamaldehyde	2.0
Eugenol	2.0
Isoeugenol	2.0
Geraniol	2.0
Oakmoss absolute	2.0
Hydroxycitronellal	2.0
Musk ambrette	1.0
Musk xylene	1.0
Musk tibetine	1.0
Musk moskene	1.0
Musk ketone	1.0
Jasmine synthetic	2.0
Benzyl salicylate	2.0
Benzyl alcohol	1.0
Vanillin	10.0
Lavender absolute	2.0
Cananga oil	2.0
Rose oil, Bulgarian	2.0
Ylang-Ylang oil	2.0
Geranium oil Bourbon	2.0
Jasmine absolute, Egyptian	2.0
Sandalwood oil	2.0

Plant Series

Chamomilla Romana (Anthemis nobilis)	1.0
Diallyl disulfide	1.0
Arnica Montana (Mountain tobacco)	0.5
Taraxacum Officinale (Dandelion)	2.5
Achillea Millefolium (Yarrow)	1.0
Propolis	10.0
Chrysanthemum Cinerariaefolium (Pyrethrum)	1.0
Sesquiterpene lactone mix	0.1
alpha-Methylene-gamma-butyrolactone	0.01
Tanacetum Vulgare (Tansy)	1.0
Alantolactone	0.1
Lichen acid mix	0.3

HERMAL/TROLAB

Perfumes, Flavors (cont'd)

Orange Oil	2
Vanillin	10
Cinnamyl Alcohol	1
Cinnamaldehyde	1
Eugenol	1
alpha-Amyl-Cinnamaldehyde	1
Hydroxycitronellal	1
Geraniol	1
Isoeugenol	1
Oak Moss Absolute	1
Benzaldehyde	5
Benzylcinnamate	5
Cedarwood Oil	10
Eucalyptus Oil	2
Laurel Oil	2
Lemon Grass Oil	2
Lemon Oil	2
Neroli Oil	2
Peppermint Oil	2
Salicylaldehyde	2

Plants, Woods

alpha-Pinene	15
Dipentene (dl-Limonene)	2
Alantolactone (Helenin)	0.1
Usnic Acid	0.1
Atranorin	0.5
Arnica Tincture	20

Tars, Balsams

Pix Lithanthracis (Coal Tar)	3
Pix Betulae (Birch Tar)	3
Pix Fagi (Beech Tar)	3
Pix Oxycedri (Juniper Tar)	3
Pix Liquida (Pine Tar)	3
Storax	2
Balsam of Pine	20
Balsam of Spruce	20
Balsam of Tolu	20
Venice Turpentine	20

CHEMOTECHNIQUE

Dental Screening

Methyl methacrylate	2.0
Triethyleneglycol dimethacrylate	2.0
Urethane dimethacrylate	2.0
Ethyleneglycol dimethacrylate	2.0
BIS-GMA	2.0
N,N-dimethyl-4-toluidine	5.0
2-Hydroxy-4-methoxybenzophenone	2.0
1, 4-Butanediol dimethacrylate	2.0
BIS-MA	2.0
Potassium dichromate	0.5
Mercury	0.5
Cobalt chloride	1.0
2-Hydroxyethyl methacrylate	2.0
Gold sodium thiosulfate	0.5
Nickel sulfate	5.0
Eugenol	2.0
Colophony	20.0
N-Ethyl-4-toluenesulfonamide	0.1
Formaldehyde	1.0
4-Tolyldiethanolamine	2.0
Copper sulfate	2.0
Methylhydroquinone	1.0
Palladium chloride	2.0
Aluminium chloride hexahydrate	2.0
Camphoroquinone	1.0
N,N-Dimethylaminoethyl methacrylate	0.2
1,6-Hexanediol diacrylate	0.1
2(2-Hydroxy-5-methylphenyl) benzotriazol	1.0
Tetrahydrofurfuryl methacrylate	2.0
Tin	50.0

HERMAL/TROLAB

Pesticides

Captan	0.1
Zineb	1
Captafol (Difolatan®)	0.1
Maneb	1
Folpet (Phaltan®)	0.1
Pyrethrum	2
Benomyl® (Benlate)	0.1
Ziram®	1

Dental Materials

Benzoyl Peroxide	1
Tetracaine Hydrochloride (Amethocaine)	1
Mercury	1
Copper Sulphate (in water)	1
Potassium Dicyanoaurate (in water)	0.002
Methyl Methacrylate	2
Hydroquinone	1
Bisphenol A	1
N,N-Dimethyl-p-Toluidine	2
Eugenol	1
Ethyleneglycol Dimethacrylate (EGDMA)	2
Triethyleneglycol Dimethacrylate (TEGDMA)	2
BIS-GMA	2

Metal Compounds

Ammoniated Mercury	1
Mercury	1
Copper Sulphate (in water)	1
Potassium Dicyanoaurate (in water)	0.002
Sodium Thiosulfatoaurate	0.5
Ammonium Tetrachloroplatinate	0.25
Palladium Chloride	1

APPENDIX 1

CHEMOTECHNIQUE

Rubber Additives Series

Tetramethylthiuram disulfide	1.0
Tetramethylthiuram monosulfide	1.0
Tetraethylthiuram disulfide	1.0
Dipentamethylenethiuram disulfide	1.0
N-Cyclohexyl-N-phenyl-4-phenylenediamine	1.0
N,N-Diphenyl-4-phenylenediamine	1.0
N-Isopropyl-N-phenyl-4-phenylenediamine	0.1
2-Mercaptobenzothiazole	2.0
N-Cyclohexylbenzothiazyl sulphenamide	1.0
Dibenzothiazyl disulfide	1.0
Morpholinylmercapto benzothiazole	1.0
Diphenylguanidine	1.0
Zinc diethyldithiocarbamate	1.0
Zinc dibutyldithiocarbamate	1.0
N,N-Di-beta-naphtyl-4-phenylenediamine	1.0
N-Phenyl-2-naphtylamine	1.0
Hexamethylenetetramine	2.0
Diaminodiphenylmethane	0.5
Diphenylthiourea	1.0
Zinc dimethyldithiocarbamate	1.0
2,2,4-Trimethyl-1,2-dihydroquinoline	1.0
Diethylthiourea	1.0
Dibutylthiourea	1.0
Dodecylmercaptan	0.1

Plastics & Glues Series

Hydroquinone	1.0
Dibutyl phtalate	5.0
Phenyl salicylate	1.0
Diethylhexylphthalate (Dioctylphthalate)	2.0
2,6-Ditert-butyl-4-cresol (BHT)	2.0
2(2-Hydroxy-5-methylphenyl)benzotriazol	1.0

HERMAL/TROLAB

Rubber Chemicals

Monobenzone (Hydroquinone Monobenzylether)	1
4,4'-Dihydroxybiphenyl	0.1
Hexamethylenetetramine	2
Dibenzothiazyl Disulphide	1
Diphenylthiourea	1
Ethylenethiourea	1
Dithiodimorpholine	1
Dibutylthiourea	1
Diethylthiourea	1
N-Cyclohexylbenzothiazyl Sulphenamide (CBS)	1
1,3-Diphenylguanidine (DPG)	1
N-Isopropyl-N'-phenyl Paraphenylenediamine (IPPD)	0.1
Tetramethylthiuram Monosulphide (TMTM)	0.25
Bis(diethyldithiocarbamato) Zinc (ZDC)	1
Tetramethylthiuram Disulphide (TMTD)	0.25
N-Cyclohexyl-N'-phenyl Paraphenylenediamine	0.25
N,N'-Diphenyl Paraphenylenediamine	0.25
Morpholinylmercaptobenzothiazole	0.5
Tetraethylthiuram Disulphide	0.25
Dipentamethylenethiuram Disulphide	0.25
Bis(dibutyldithiocarbamato) Zinc	1
Piperazine	1
Cyclohexyl Thiophthalimide	1

Plastics, Glues

Phenol Formaldehyde Resin, Novolac	5
Triethylenetetramine	0.5
4,4'-Diaminodiphenyl Methane	0.5
Toluenesulphonamide Formaldehyde Resin	10
Urea Formaldehyde Resin	10
Melamine Formaldehyde Resin	10

CHEMOTECHNIQUE

Plastics & Glues Series (cont'd)

Benzoylperoxide	1.0
4-tert.Butylcatechol (PTBC)	0.5
Azodiisobutyrodinitrile	1.0
Bisphenol A	1.0
Tricresyl phosphate	5.0
Phenol formaldehyde resin (P-F-R-2)	1.0
p-tert-Butylphenol formaldehyde resin	1.0
Triphenyl phosphate	5.0
Toluenesulfonamide formaldehyde resin	10.0
Resorcinol monobenzoate	1.0
2-Phenylindole	2.0
2-tert-Butyl-4-methoxyphenol (BHA)	2.0
Abitol	10.0
4-tert-Butylphenol	1.0
2-Monomethylol phenol	1.0
Diphenyl thiourea	1.0
2-n-Octyl-4-isothiazolin-3-one	0.1
Cyclohexanone resin	1.0
Triglycidyl isocyanurate	0.5

Epoxy Series

Hexamethylenetetramine	2.0
Diaminodiphenylmethane	0.5
Triethylenetetramine	0.5
Phenylglycidylether	0.25
Diethylenetriamine	1.0
Isophorone diamine	0.1
Epoxy resin, cycloaliphatic	0.5
Ethylenediamine dihydrochloride	1.0

HERMAL/TROLAB

Plastics, Glues (cont'd)

Phenol Formaldehyde Resin, Resol	5
Resorcinol Monobenzoate	1
Diethylenetriamine	0.5
Isophoronediamine	0.5
Abitol	10
alpha-Pinene	15
Cresylglycidylether	0.25
Paratertiary Butylcatechol	1
Paratertiary Butylphenol	2
Benzoyl Peroxide	1
Turpentine Oil	10
Di-n-Butylphthalate	5
Tricresyl Phosphate	5
n-Butylglycidylether	0.25
Phenylglycidylether	0.25
Diethylphthalate	5
Diisodecylphthalate	5
Dimethylphthalate	5
Diphenylmethane 4,4-Diisocyanate	0.1
Phenylisocyanate	0.1
Toluenediisocyanate	0.1
Triphenylmethane Triisocyanate	0.1
Triphenyl Phosphate	5
Di-2-Ethylhexyl-Phthalate	5
Butyl Acrylate	0.1
Epichlorohydrin	0.1
N,N-Dimethyl-p-Toluidine	2
Abietic Acid	5
Bisphenol A	1

CHEMOTECHNIQUE HERMAL/TROLAB

Isocyanate Series

Toluenediisocyanate (TDI)	2.0
Diphenylmethane-4,4-diisocyanate (MDI)	2.0
Diaminodiphenylmethane	0.5
Isophoronediisocyanate (IPDI)	1.0
Isophorone diamine (IPD)	0.1
1,6-Hexamethylenediisocyanate (HDI)	0.1

(Meth) Acrylate Series
Adhesives, Dental & Other

Methyl methacrylate	2.0
n-Butyl methacrylate	2.0
2-Hydroxyethyl methacrylate	2.0
2-Hydroxypropyl methacrylate	2.0
Ethyleneglycol dimethacrylate	2.0
Triethyleneglycol dimethacrylate	2.0
1,4-Butanediol dimethacrylate	2.0
Urethane dimethacrylate	2.0
BIS-MA	2.0
BIS-GMA	2.0
1,6-Hexanediol diacrylate	0.1
Tetrahydrofurfuryl methacrylate	2.0
Tetraethyleneglycol dimethacrylate	2.0
N,N-Dimethylaminoethyl methacrylate	0.2

(Meth) Acrylate Series
Nails—Artificial

Butyl acrylate	0.1
Ethyl methacrylate	2.0
n-Butyl methacrylate	2.0
2-Hydroxyethyl methacrylate	2.0
2-Hydroxypropyl methacrylate	2.0
Ethyleneglycol dimethacrylate	2.0
Triethyleneglycol dimethacrylate	2.0
1,6-Hexanediol diacrylate	0.1
Trimethylolpropane triacrylate	0.1

CHEMOTECHNIQUE

(Meth) Acrylate Series (cont'd)
Nails—Artificial

Tetrahydrofurfuryl methacrylate	2.0
Ethyl acrylate	0.1
2-Hydroxyethyl acrylate	0.1
Triethyleneglycol diacrylate	0.1

(Meth) Acrylate Series
Printing

Ethyl acrylate	0.1
2-Ethylhexyl acrylate	0.1
2-Hydroxyethyl acrylate	0.1
2-Hydroxypropyl acrylate	0.1
Methyl methacrylate	2.0
Ethyl methacrylate	2.0
n-Butyl methacrylate	2.0
2-Hydroxyethyl methacrylate	2.0
2-Hydroxypropyl methacrylate	2.0
Ethyleneglycol dimethacrylate	2.0
Triethyleneglycol dimethacrylate	2.0
BIS-EMA	1.0
1,4-Butanediol diacrylate	0.1
1,6-Hexanediol diacrylate	0.1
Diethyleneglycol diacrylate	0.1
Tripropyleneglycol diacrylate	0.1
Trimethylolpropane triacrylate	0.1
Pentaerythritol triacrylate	0.1
Oligotriacrylate 480	0.1
Epoxy acrylate	0.5
Urethane diacrylate (aliphatic)	0.1
Urethane diacrylate (aromatic)	0.05
Triethyleneglycol diacrylate	0.1
N,N-Methylenebisacrylamid	1.0

Photographic Chemicals Series

CD-2	1.0
CD-3	1.0
CD-4	1.0
4-Methylaminophenol sulfate (Metol)	1.0
Hydroquinone	1.0

HERMAL/TROLAB

Photographic Chemicals

Ammonium Persulphate	2.5
p-Methylaminophenol Sulphate (Metol)	1
Color Developer CD 2	1
Color Developer CD 3	1
Color Developer CD 1	1

APPENDIX 1

CHEMOTECHNIQUE

Photographic Chemicals Series (cont'd)

Phenidone	1.0
Hydroxylammonium chloride	0.1
Ammoniumpersulfate	2.5
Ethylenediamine dihydrochloride	1.0
1H-Benzotriazol	1.0
Glutaraldehyde	0.2
Benzylalcohol	1.0
Hydroxylammonium sulfate	0.1
Potassium dichromate	0.5
4-Amino-N,N-diethylaniline sulfate (TSS)	1.0
Tricresyl phosphate	5.0

Oil & Cooling Fluid Series

Abietic acid	10.0
4-Chloro-3-cresol (PCMC)	1.0
4-Chloro-3-xylenol (PCMX)	0.5
Dichlorophene	1.0
2-Phenylphenol	1.0
Propyleneglycol	5.0
Triethanolamine	2.0
4-tert-Butylbenzoic acid	1.0
1,2-Benzisothiazolin-3-one	0.05
Hexahydro-1,3,5-tris (hydroxyethyl) triazin	1.0
Bioban P 1487	0.5
Chloroacetamide	0.2
N-Methylol chloroacetamide	0.1
1H-Benzotriazol	1.0
Ethylenediamine dihydrochloride	1.0
Mercaptobenzothiazole	2.0
Zinc ethylenebis (dithiocarbamate)	1.0
Triclosan (Irgasan DP 300)	2.0
Bioban CS 1246	1.0
Bioban CS 1135	1.0
Tris nitro	1.0
Thimerosal (Merthiolate)	0.1
Hydrazine sulfate	1.0
Trichlorocarbanilide (TCC)	1.0
Formaldehyde	1.0
Amerchol L 101	100

HERMAL/TROLAB

Photographic Chemicals (cont'd)

Color Developer CD 4	1
Color Developer CD 32	1
Color Developer CD 60	1
1-Phenyl-3-pyrazolidinone (Phenidone)	1
Pyrogallol	1
p-Aminophenol	2
Hydroquinone	1
Hydrazine Sulphate	1
Pyrocatechol	2
Triphenyl Phosphate	5

CHEMOTECHNIQUE

Oil & Cooling Fluid Series (cont'd)

Dipentene (Limonene)	1.0
Sodium-2-pyridinethiol-1-oxide	0.1
2-Bromo-2-nitropropane-1,3-diol	0.25
Coconut diethanolamide	0.5
Cl + Me-isothiazolinone (Kathon CG,200ppm)	1.34
Euxyl K 400	0.5
2-n-Octyl-4-isothiazolin-3-one	0.1

Textile Colours & Finish

Disperse Yellow 3	1.0
Disperse Orange 3	1.0
Disperse Red 1	1.0
Disperse Red 17	1.0
Disperse Blue 153	1.0
Disperse Blue 3	1.0
Disperse Blue 35	1.0
Dimethylol dihydroxyethyleneurea (Fix.CPN)	4.5
Dimethylol propylene urea (Fix.PH)	5.0
Tetramethylol acetylenediurea (Fix.140)	5.0
Disperse Blue 106	1.0
Ethyleneurea, melamineformaldehyde (Fix.Ac)	5.0
Urea formaldehyde (Kaurit S)	10.0
Melamine formaldehyde (Kaurit M70)	7.0
Disperse Blue 85	1.0
Disperse Orange 1	1.0
Disperse Orange 13	1.0
Disperse Brown 1	1.0
Disperse Yellow 9	1.0
Disperse Blue 124	1.0
Basic Red 46	1.0

Shoe Series

N-Isopropyl-N-phenyl-4-phenylenediamine	0.1
Glutaraldehyde	1.0

HERMAL/TROLAB

Textile Finishes

Urea Formaldehyde Resin	10
Melamine Formaldehyde Resin	10

Organic Dyes

Disperse Orange 3	1
Disperse Yellow 3	1
Disperse Red 1	1
Disperse Red 17	1
Disperse Blue 3	1
Eosine	50
p-Aminophenol	2

CHEMOTECHNIQUE

HERMAL/TROLAB

Shoe Series (cont'd)

Disperse Orange 3	1.0
Acid Yellow 36	1.0
Hydroquinone monobenzylether	1.0
Thiuram mix	1.0
Potassium dichromate	0.5
4-tert-Butylphenol formaldehyde resin	1.0
4-Phenylenediamine base	1.0
Nickel sulfate	5.0
Colophony	20.0
Formaldehyde	1.0
Diphenyl thiourea	1.0
2-Mercaptobenzothiazole	2.0
Diethylthiourea	1.0
Diphenylguanidine	1.0
Dibutylthiourea	1.0
Epoxy resin	1.0
Dodecylmercaptan	0.1
Cl + Me-isothiazolinone (Kathon CG, 200 ppm)	1.34
4-Aminoazobenzene	0.25
2-n-Octyl-4-isothiazolin-3-one	0.1

Bakery Series

Vanillin	10.0
Eugenol	2.0
Isoeugenol	2.0
Sodium benzoate	5.0
2, 6-Ditert-butyl-4-cresol (BHT)	2.0
Menthol	2.0
Cinnamic alcohol	2.0
Cinnamic aldehyde	1.0
2-tert-Butyl-4-methoxyphenol (BHA)	2.0
Anethole	5.0
Sorbic acid	2.0
Benzoic acid	5.0
Propionic acid	3.0
Octyl gallate	0.25
Dipentene (Limonene)	1.0
Ammonium persulfate	2.5
Benzoylperoxide	1.0
Propyl gallate	1.0
Dodecyl gallate	0.25

CHEMOTECHNIQUE

Scandinavian Photo Patch

Trichlorcarbanilide (TCC)	1.0
Promethazine hydrochloride	1.0
4-Aminobenzoic acid (PABA)	5.0
Tribromsalicylanilide (TBS)	1.0
Chlorpromazine hydrochloride	0.1
Musk ambrette	1.0
6-Methylcoumarine (6-MC)	1.0
Bithionol	1.0
Fentichlor	1.0
D-Usnic acid	0.1
Atranorin	0.1
Wood mix (pine, spruce, birch, teak)	20.0
Evernic acid	0.1
Balsam Peru	25.0
Tetrachlorsalicylanilide (TCS)	0.1
Hexachlorophene	1.0
Chlorhexidine digluconate	0.5
Triclosan (Irgasan DP 300)	2.0
Diphenhydramine hydrochloride	1.0
Perfume mix	6.0

HERMAL/TROLAB

Photoallergens

Tribromsalan	1
6-Methylcoumarin	1
Chlorpromazine Hydrochloride	0.1
Fenticlor	1
Musk Ambrette	5
Promethazine Hydrochloride	1
p-Aminobenzoic Acid (PABA)	5
Bithionol	1
Hexachlorophene	1
Tetrachloro Salicylanilide	0.1
Chlorhexidine (Diacetate (in water)	0.5
Diphenydramine Hydrochloride	1
Moskene	5
Musk Ketone	5
Musk Xylene	5
Thiourea	0.1
Triclocarban	1

MAILING ADDRESSES

Chemotechnique Diagnostic AB
Ringugnsgatan 7
S-216 16 Malmö, Sweden
Tel: (46-40) 160236
Fax: (46-40) 158640

Hermal Kurt Herrmann
P.O. Box 12 28, D-2057 Reinbek/Hamburg, Germany
Tel: 40-72704-0
Fax: 40-7229296

Distributed in North America by:

Dormer Laboratories, Inc.
6600 Trans Canada Highway, Suite 750
Pointe-Claire, Quebec, H9R 4S2
Tel: 514-697-0519
Fax: 514-451-6685

Pharmascience Inc. (Omniderm)
8400 ch. Darnley Rd.
CND—Montréal, Québec H4T 1M4
Tel: 514-340-11 14, Telex: 05-824 588 pms mtl, Fax: 001/514 342 7764

Hermal Imported and distributed in:

Australia and New Zealand:
W.E. & M. Schroeder,
P.O. Box 11
AUS—Thornleigh, 2120 N.S.W.
Tel: 02-481-09 27, Telex: AA 21730,
Fax: 612 875 2857

Chile:
Promedar Ltda.
Barros Borgoño 297
RCH—Santiago
Tel: 2 23 28 58, Telex: 240 301, Telefax: 56-2-2322587

Finland:
Oy Tamro Ab
PB 11
SF—01641 Vantaa
Tel: 358-0-852 011, Telefax: 358-0-85 20 1010

France:
Laboratories PROMEDICA
7 Avenue Pasteur
F—92400 Courbevoie
Tel: (1) 47 68 88 99, Telex: 613050 prome f
Telefax: (1) 43 34 02 79

Great Britain and the Republic of Ireland:
Bio Diagnostics Ltd.
Upton Industrial Estate,
Rectory Road,
Upton upon Severn
GB-Worcestershire WR8 OXL
Tel: 0 684-59 22 62, Telefax: 0 68 4-59 25 01

Hongkong:
Jebsen & Co. Ltd.
9/F1, Scomber Building
1 Yip Fat Street
Wong Chuk Hang
HK—Hongkong
Tel: 8737070, Telefax: 8459069, 8681742

Israel:
Neopharm Ltd., P.O. Box 7108
IL—Tel-Aviv 61070
Tel: 972-3-56 27 777, Telex: 342175 neopm il, Telefax: 972-3-56 26 080

Italy:
Bracco Industria Chimica s.p.a., Via Egidio Folli 50
I—20134 Milano
Tel: 02-2177321/2, Telex: 311185 bracco i, Telefax: 02/264 10678

Malaysia:
Germax Sdn. Bhd.
P.O. Box 6514 Kampung Tunku,
MAL—47307 Petaling Jaya
Selangor Darul Ehsan
Tel: 776 13 45/776 13 88, Telex: 37455 berkat ma Telefax: 03-775 58 79

The Netherlands, Belgium, Luxembourg:
van der Bend B. V.,
P.O. Box 73
NL—3230 AB Brielle
Tel: 0 18 10-18 055, Telefax: 0 18 10-17 450

Norway:
Merck AIS
P.O. Box 51
Ellingsrudasen
N—1006 Oslo 10
Tel: (02) 32 11 50, Telex: 77 413 mas n, Telefax: (02) 30 52 44

Portugal:
Laboratório Fidelis, Lda.
Apartado 180
P—2795 Linda-a-Velha Codex
Tel: 410 20 77, Telex: 12042 fideli p,
Telefax: 0035-114106345

Singapore:
Wellchem Pharmaceuticals (Pte.) Ltd.
Blk. 36 H, No. 02—46, Chancery Court, Dunearn Road
SGP—Singapore 1130
Tel: 253 45 33, Telefax: 65—25 42 720

Sweden:
E. Merck AB
Kungsgatan 65
S—11122 Stockholm
Tel: 08-23 36 85, Telex: 10677, Telefax: (08) 24 55 94

Thailand:
B. Grimm & Co. R.O.P.
G.P.O. Box 66
1643/4 Phetburi Rd.
T—Bangkok 10310
Tel: (622) 252-4081, 252-9131
Telex: 82614 bgrim th., Telefax: 2539867

Turkey:
MEDSAN ITHALAT & IHRACAT
ILAÇ SAN. VE TIC. LTD. STI.
Yakitçilar sk. 6/7 Sihhiye
TR—Ankara
Tel: (4) 134 21 40
Telefax: (4) 134 21 44

Appendix 2

Chemical Resistance Charts for Work and General Gloves Available From:

Ansell Edmont Industrial
1300 Walnut Street
Box 6000
Coshocton, Ohio 43812-6000
Tel: 1-800-800-0444
Fax: 1-800-800-0455

North Hand Protection
A Division of Siebe North, Inc.
P.O. Box 70729
Charleston, South Carolina 29415
Tel: 803-745-5900
Fax: 803-744-2857

In Canada
North Safety Products
25 Dansk Court
Rexdale, Ontario
Canada, M9W 5V8
Tel: 416-675-2810
Fax: 416-675-6898

Appendix 3

Hypoallergic Gloves and Products Available From:

Allerderm
Allerderm Laboratories, Inc.
P.O. Box 2070
Petaluma, California 94953-2070
Tel: 1-800-365-6868
Fax: 1-800-926-4568

The Skin & Allergy Shop
310 East Broadway
Louisville, Kentucky 40202
Tel: 1-800-366-6483
Fax: 502-589-3429

Appendix 4

Common Latex Examination Gloves and Their Associated Antigens[1,2]

Gloves	Manufacturer	MBT	TH	CAR	LOW	BHA	ST	GI	Comments
Surgeon's latex gloves									
Bio Gel D	Reagent Hospital Products, Mamoroneck, NY	–	–	+	–	–	–	+	Powder-free, low in CAR
Eudermic	Beckton Dickinson, Franklin Lakes, N.J.	–	–	+	NA	NA	+	+	Latex
Medigrip	Ansell	+	+	+	–	–	+	+	
Micro-Touch	Surgikos, Arlington, Tex.	+	–	+	–	–	+	+	White or brown latex
Neutralon	Surgikos	+	–	+	–	–	+	+	Polyurethane elastomer; patented; inner coating brown glove
Perry Derma-Guard	Smith & Nephew Medical, Massillon, Ohio	+	–	+	+	–	+	+	Brown glove
Perry Standard	Smith & Nephew Medical	+	+	+	+	–	+	+	White or brown latex
Pristine	World Medical Supply, San Jose, Calif.	–	+	–	–	–	–	+	Powder-free; dipenta-methylenethiuram tetrasulfide
Puritée	Orox, Cincinnati, Ohio	–	–	–	–	+	+	+	Pure rubber; powder is optional; packet is included
Sensi-Touch	Ansell	+	–	+	–	–	+	+	
Travenol	Baxter Pharmaseal, Valencia, Calif.	+	–	+	–	–	+	+	
Ultraderm	Baxter Pharmaseal	–	–	+	–	–	+	+	Low CAR

Product	Manufacturer							Comments
Surgeon's synthetic gloves								
Dermaprene	Ansell, Dothan, Ala.	−	−	−	−	+	+	Neoprene; accelerator isodiphenylthiourea; green
Elastyren	Allerderm Labs, Calif.	−	−	+	−	+	+	Styrene butadiene block polymer; available in sterile and nonsterile
Neolon	Becton Dickinson	−	−	+	−	−	+	Neoprene glove; low in CAR lactose powder; brown glove
Vinyl examining gloves								
TriFlex	Baxter Pharmaseal	−	−	−	−	+	−	Available in sterile and nonsterile; sterilized with ethylene oxide
TruTouch	Becton Dickinson	−	−	−	−	+	−	Available in sterile and nonsterile; sterilized with ethylene oxide
Surgikos	Surgikos	−	−	−	−	+	+	Available sterile or nonsterile
Latex examining gloves								
Flexam Exam	Baxter Pharmaseal	+	−	+	++	+	+	Produced in Malaysia; both sterile and nonsterile available
Flexam Exam	Baxter Pharmaseal	++	+	++	++	+	+	Domestically produced; both sterile and nonsterile available
Medigrip	Ansell, Inc.	++	−	++	−	++	−	
Perry orthopedic	Smith & Nephew Medical	+	+	++	−	++	+	Thicker than Perry examination glove
Perry sterile examination	Smith & Nephew Medical	+	+	+	−	+	+	Available in both sterile and nonsterile
Sensi-Touch	Ansell	+	+	−	−	+	−	Nonsterile examination glove

161

		Antigen							
Gloves	Manufacturer	MBT	TH	CAR	LOW	BHA	ST	GI	Comments
Travenol	Baxter Pharmaseal	+	–	+	–	–	+	+	
Travenol procedure	Baxter Pharmaseal	+	–	+	–	–	+	+	Available in right- and left-handed gloves
Household weight gloves									
Allerderm cotton	Allerderm Lab	–	–	–	–	–	–	–	Cotton; can be used as glove liner; can order directly from company
Allerderm vinyl	Allerderm Lab	–	–	–	–	–	–	–	Vinyl glove that contains mica powder; can be ordered direct from company
Bluette Benchmarks	Pioneer Consumer Glove Willard, Ohio	–	–	+	–	–	–	–	Neoprene lined with knitted cotton; talc used in manufacturing
Nimble-fingers	Pioneer Consumer Glove	–	–	–	–	–	–	–	Vinyl pylox (light weight); contains mica powder; no accelerators used
Task Handlers	Pioneer Consumer Glove	–	–	–	–	–	–	–	Neoprene; *does* contain CaCO$_3$ powder
4H	Acaderm, Menlo Park, Calif.	NA	NA	NA	NA	NA	–	–	Patented; plastic laminate

CAR, Carbamates; *GI*, gamma irradiation sterilization; *LOW*, Lowinox 44S36; *MBT*, mercaptobenzothiazole; *NA*, information not available; *ST*, starch powder; *TH*, tetramethylthiuram.
1. Rich P, Belozer ML, Norris P, et al: Allergic contact dermatitis to two antioxidants in latex gloves: 4,4′-thiobis(6-tert-butyl-meta-cresol) (Lowinox 44S36) and butylhydroxyanisole. J Am Acad Dermatol 24:37–43, 1991.
2. Storrs FJ: Allergic contact dermatitis to latex glove antioxidants: an update. J Am Acad Dermatol 26:144, 1992.

Appendix 5

Addresses of societies for dermatologists interested in contact dermatitis and occupational dermatoses:

American Contact Dermatitis Society
930 N. Meacham Road
Schaumburg, Illinois 60173-6016
Tel: (708) 330-9830
Fax: (708) 330-0050

European Society of Contact Dermatitis
Dr. Derk P. Bruynzeel
Treasurer, ESCD
Department of Occupational Dermatology
Free University Academic Hospital
De Boelelaan 1117
NL-1081 HV Amsterdam
The Netherlands

Addresses of the societies' journals:

American Journal of Contact Dermatitis
W.B. Saunders Company
Periodicals Department
6277 Sea Harbor Drive
Orlando, Florida 32887-4800

Contact Dermatitis
MUNKSGAARD International Publishers Ltd.
35 Nerre Sogade
Postbox 2148
DK-1016 Copenhagen K, Denmark
Tel: +4533127030
Fax: +4533129387

MUNKSGAARD International
Publishers Ltd.
238 Main Street
Cambridge, Massachusetts
02142-9740
Tel: (617) 547-7665
Fax: (617) 545-7489

Index

A
Acids, irritant contact dermatitis, 6
Acne, 18, 90–92
  chloracne, 90–92
  coal tar-induced, 90
  diagnosis, 36–37
  environmental halogen acne, 90–92
  petroleum-induced, 90
Adhesive, patch testing, 62
Adjuster, insurance company, report to, 124–128
Adverse reactions, patch testing, 51
Aggravation, defined, 130
Al-Test chamber, 44–45
Alkalis, irritant contact dermatitis, 7
Allergic contact dermatitis
  balsam of Peru, 9
  benzocaine, 11
  black rubber mix, 10
  carbamates, 9–10
  colophony, 11
  epoxy resin, 8
  ethylenediamine, 11
  formaldehyde, 9
  imidazolidinyl urea, 9
  lanolin alcohol, 11
  mercapto mix, 10
  mercaptobenzothiazole, 9
  neomycin sulfate, 11
  nickel sulfate, 11
  nonoccupational origin, diagnosis, 34
  occupational groups, 7–12
  para-tertiary-butylphenol, 8–9
  paraphenylenediamine, 8
  potassium dichromate, 10
  quaternium 15, 9
  regional distribution, 5
  rosin, 11
  thiuram mix, 10
  treatment, 108–109
Allergen series, for specific occupations, 66–68
Antibiotics, for occupational dermatitis, 106
Antimicrobials, patch testing, 61–63
Arsenic, inorganic, skin cancer, 94–95
Asteatotic eczema, diagnosis, 35
Athletic shoes, patch testing, 79
Atopic/dyshidrotic eczema, diagnosis, 35
Atopic eczema, diagnosis, 35

B
Bacterial infection, 96–97
Bakery series, patch testing, 67
Balsam of Peru
  allergic contact dermatitis, 9
  patch testing, 65
Banker, patch testing, 78
Barrier cream, 105
  versus chromate, for hand eczema, 110
Benzocaine
  allergic contact dermatitis, 11
  patch testing, 64
Benzoyl peroxide, irritant contact dermatitis, 7
Biocides, patch testing, 61–63

Black rubber mix
  allergic contact dermatitis, 10
  patch testing, 60
Bleach, irritant contact dermatitis, 7
Board, workers' compensation, 129–140

C

Cancer, skin, 93–96
  arsenic, inorganic, 94–95
  ionizing radiation, 95
  malignant melanoma, 95–96
  polycyclic hydrocarbons, 94
  ultraviolet light, 95
Carba mix, patch testing, 60
Carbamates, allergic contact dermatitis, 9–10
Chef, patch testing, 72
Chemotechnique, 155
  patch testing, 68
Chloracne, 90–92
Cinnamic aldehyde
  allergic contact dermatitis, 7–8
  patch testing, 65
Cleansers, irritant contact dermatitis, 6
Clerical worker, patch testing, 78
Coal tar-induced acne, 90
Colophony
  allergic contact dermatitis, 11
  patch testing, 62
Commercial trays, for patch tests, 142–155
Compensability, defined, 130
Construction workers, patch testing, 75
Contact dermatitis
  allergic, see Allergic contact dermatitis
  exogenous, see Exogenous contact dermatitis
  irritant, see Irritant contact dermatitis
Contact urticaria, 81–88
  causes, 83–86
  controls, testing, 86
  defined, 81–82
  diagnosis, 34, 82–83
  from latex protein, 87
  symptoms, 82
Cook, patch testing, 72
Corrective action, occupational dermatitis, 118
Cosmetician, patch testing, 75–77
Cosmetics, irritant contact dermatitis, 15
Credibility, see Terminology
Cutting fluid series, patch testing, 67

D

Dapsone, for hand eczema, 109
Data sheet, material safety, sample, 120–121
Delusional belief, of parasitosis, 38
Dental series, patch testing, 67
Dermal reticulosis, diagnosis, 32–33
Dermatitis, defined, 2
Dermatoheliosis, diagnosis, 34
Desiccants, irritant contact dermatitis, 14–15
Detergents, irritant contact dermatitis, 6
Diagnosis
  acneiform eruptions, 36–37
  allergic contact dermatitis of nonoccupational origin, 34
  asteatotic eczema, 35
  atopic/dyshidrotic eczema, 35
  contact urticaria, 34, 82–83
  dermal reticulosis, 32–33
  dermatoheliosis, 34
  dyshidrotic eczema, 35
  eczema/dermatitis, 33–34
  endogenous eczema, 35–36
  epoxy resin exposure, 27
  exogenous eczema/dermatoses, 33–34
  ichthyoses, 33
  impetigo, 27
  infectious dermatoses, 36–37
  irritant contact dermatitis, 18–20
  irritant dermatitis, 33–34
  keratodermas, 36
  lichen planus, 32
  Münchausen's syndrome, 38
  nonoccupational dermatoses, 29–38
  occupational dermatoses, 24–40
  papulosquamous dermatoses, 29–33
  pigmentary disorder, 38
  psoriasiform keratoderma, 25
  psoriasis, 29–31
  seborrheic dermatitis, 35–36
  Secretan's syndrome, 38
  tinea manuum, 32
  vesicobullous disease, 37
  xerotic eczema, 35
Dietary modification, for hand eczema, 109
Disability, defined, 130
Disabling claim, defined, 130
Dyshidrotic eczema, diagnosis, 35

E

Eczema, hand
  dapsone, 109
  nickel allergy, novel therapy, 109
  novel therapy, 109–110
Eczema/dermatitis, diagnosis, 33–34
Emollients, for occupational dermatitis, 106–107
Endogenous eczema, diagnosis, 35–36
Environmental factors, irritant contact dermatitis, 16
Environmental halogen acne, 90–92

INDEX

Epiquick, patch testing, 44
Epoxy resin
    allergic contact dermatitis, 8
    exposure, diagnosis, 27
    patch testing, 64
Estheticians, patch testing, 75–77
Ethylenediamine
    allergic contact dermatitis, 11
    patch testing, 65
European Standard Tray, patch testing, 47
Exogenous contact dermatitis, 2–3
Exogenous eczema/dermatoses, diagnosis, 33–34
Exposure factors, irritant contact dermatitis, 16

F

False patch testing reading, 49–50
Fingernail changes, 100
Finn chamber, 44–46
Flavorings, patch testing, 65
Florists, patch testing, 72–75
Food handlers, patch testing, 72
Formaldehyde
    allergic contact dermatitis, 9
    patch testing, 62, 77–78
Fragrances, patch testing, 65
Friction irritant contact dermatitis, 18
Functionelle Hautprufung, contact test, 41
Fungus, 97–98

G

Gardeners, patch testing, 72–75
Glove
    protective, in treatment, 105–106
    rubber, 2, 158–162
        psoriasiform keratoderma, 25
Gourmet cooks, patch testing, 72

H

Hairdressers, patch testing, 75–77
Hairdressing series, patch testing, 67
Hand, eczema
    barrier cream versus chromate, 110
    dapsone, 109
    dietary modification, 109
    nickel allergy, novel therapy, 109
    novel therapy, 109–110
Hand washing, as treatment, for occupational dermatitis, 106
Health care workers, patch testing, 71–72
Hermal patch test, 44
Host factors, irritant contact dermatitis, 16
Humidity, reaction to, 99

Hydrogen peroxide, irritant contact dermatitis, 7
Hyperpigmentation, 92–93
Hypopigmentation, pigmentary disorder, 93

I

Ichthyoses, diagnosis, 33
Imidazolidinyl urea, allergic contact dermatitis, 9
Impairment, defined, 130
Impetigo, 27
Industrial hygiene terminology, 118–123
Industrial setting, irritants in, 20
Infection, 96–98
    bacteria, 96–97
    fungi, 97–98
    parasite, 98
    virus, 96
Infectious dermatoses, diagnosis, 36–37
Insurance company, report to, 124–128
Interpretation, patch testing results, 50–51
Ionizing radiation, skin cancer, 95
Irritant contact dermatitis, 3–7, 13–23
    acids, 6
    acneiform, 18
    acute, 16–17
    alkalis, 7
    benzoyl peroxide, 7
    bleach, 7
    cleansers, 6
    clinical presentation, 16–18
    cosmetics, 15
    cumulative, 17
    delayed, acute, 17
    desiccants, 14–15
    detergents, 6
    diagnostic criteria, 18–20
    environmental factors, 16
    exposure factors, 16
    friction irritation, 18
    host factors, 16
    hydrogen peroxide, 7
    irritant reaction, 17
    lubricants, 6
    nonerythematous irritation, 18
    occupational groups, 5–7
    oils, 6
    oxidizing agent, 7
    pathophysiology, 13
    plant products, 7
    prevention, 20–21
    prognosis, 21
    pustular, 18
    reducing agent, 7
    sensitization, vs. irritation, 13
    therapy, 21

Irritant contact dermatitis (contd.)
    thioglycolates, 7
    traumatic, 17–18
    treatment, 107–108
    types of irritants, 14–15
    water, 5
Irritant dermatitis, diagnosis, 33–34
Irritants, types of, 14–15
Irritation, vs. sensitization, 13
Isocyanate series, patch testing, 67

K
Keratodermas, diagnosis, 36
Knitters, patch testing, 77–78

L
Lanolin alcohol, allergic contact dermatitis, 11
Latex protein, *see also* Rubber gloves
    contact urticaria, 87
Latex rubber, contact dermatitis, 2, 158–162
Legal issues, occupational exposure, 116
Lichen planus, diagnosis, 32
Light, ultraviolet, skin cancer, 95
Lubricants, irritant contact dermatitis, 6

M
Malignant melanoma, skin cancer, 95–96
Material safety data sheet, sample, 120–121
Materials, for patch testing, 42–44, 141–143
Medically stationary, defined, 130–131
Medications, topical, patch testing, 64–65
Mercapto mix
    allergic contact dermatitis, 10
    patch testing, 60
Mercaptobenzothiazole
    allergic contact dermatitis, 9
    patch testing, 55, 60
Metal allergens, patch testing, 61
Münchausen's syndrome, 38

N
Nail changes, 100
Neomycin, patch testing, 64
Neomycin sulfate, allergic contact dermatitis, 11
Newspaper writers, patch testing, 78
Nickel
    allergic contact dermatitis, 11
    allergy, hand eczema, novel therapy, 109
    patch testing, 61

North American Contact Dermatitis Group, standard allergens, 141
Nurserymen, patch testing, 72–75

O
Occupational disease, defined, 131
Occupational groups
    allergic contact dermatitis, 7–12
    irritant contact dermatitis, 5–7
Occupational injury, defined, 131
Oils, irritant contact dermatitis, 6
Oxidizing agent, irritant contact dermatitis, 7

P
p-Phenylenediamine, allergic contact dermatitis, 8
p-Phenylenediamine, patch testing, 65
p-tert-butylphenol formaldehyde resin, patch testing, 64
Paper, contact with, patch testing, 78
Papulosquamous dermatoses, diagnosis, 29–33
Para-tertiary-butylphenol, allergic contact dermatitis, 8–9
Parasites, 98
Parasitosis, delusional belief of, 38
Patch testing, 41–53
    adhesive, 62
    adverse reactions, 51
    Al-Test chamber, 44–45
    allergens, 46–50
    allergens not in standard tray, 70–80, 141–143
    antimicrobials, 61–63
    athletic shoes, 79
    bakery series, 67
    balsam of Peru, 65
    banker, 78
    benzocaine, 64
    biocides, 61–63
    black rubber mix, 60
    carba mix, 60
    chefs, 72
    Chemotechnique, 155
    cinnamic aldehyde, 65
    clerical worker, 78
    colophony, 62
    commercial patch test trays, 142–155
    construction workers, 75
    cosmeticians, 75–77
    cutting fluid series, 67
    dental series, 67
    Epiquick, 44
    epoxy resin, 64

estheticians, 75–77
ethylenediamine dihydrochloride, 65
European Standard Tray, 47
false test reading, 49–50
finding allergens in workplace, 66
Finn chamber, 44–46
flavorings, 65
florists, 72–75
food handlers, 72
formaldehyde, 62, 77–78
fragrances, 65
functionelle Hautprufung, contact test, 41
gardeners, 72–75
gourmet cooks, 72
hairdressers, 75–77
hairdressing series, 67
health care workers, 71–72
Hermal, 44
isocyanate series, 67
knitters, 77–78
lanolin, 65
materials, 42–44
mercapto mix, 60
mercaptobenzothiazole, 55, 60
metal allergens, 61
morphology codes, 141
neomycin, 64
newspaper writers, 78
nickel, 61
nurserymen, 72–75
p-phenylenediamine, 65
p-tert-butylphenol formaldehyde resin, 64
paper, contact with, 78
patient selection, 42
photographic series, 67
plastic, 62
plastic series, 67
potassium dichromate, 61
preservatives, 61–63
procedures, 42–44
result interpretation, 50–51
rubber additive series, 67
rubber allergens, 55, 60
scoring, 48
seamstresses, 77–78
specific occupations, allergen series for, 66–68
standard screening sets, 54–69
  allergens not in, 70–80, 141–143
supply sources, 52, 141–143
tape, 44
test application, 44–46
test system, 44
textile colors/finish series, 67, 141–143
textile dye, 77–78
textile workers, 77–78

thiuram mix, 60
topical medications, 64–65
True test, 44, 157
wool alcohol, 65
Patient selection, patch testing, 42
Permanency, defined, 131
Petroleum-induced acne, 90
Photographic series, patch testing, 67
Pigmentary disorder, 92–93
  diagnosis, 38
  hyperpigmentation, 92–93
  hypopigmentation, 93
Plant products, irritant contact dermatitis, 7
Plastic, patch testing, 62
Plastic series, patch testing, 67
Polycyclic hydrocarbons, skin cancer, 94
Potassium dichromate
  allergic contact dermatitis, 10
  patch testing, 61
Preservatives, patch testing, 61–63
Psoriasiform keratoderma, 25
Psoriasis, diagnosis, 29–31
Pustular irritant contact dermatitis, 18

Q
Quaternium 15, allergic contact dermatitis, 9

R
Radiation, ionizing, skin cancer, 95
Reading, false, patch test, 49–50
Reasonable medical probability, defined, 131
Reducing agent, irritant contact dermatitis, 7
Report, to insurance company, 124–128
Reticulosis, dermal, diagnosis, 32–33
Rosin, allergic contact dermatitis, 11
Rubber additive series, patch testing, 67
Rubber allergens, patch testing, 55, 60
Rubber glove, *see* Glove, rubber

S
Scheduled injury, defined, 131
Scleroderma, 99–100
Scoring patch test, 48
Seamstresses, patch testing, 77–78
Seborrheic dermatitis, diagnosis, 35–36
Secretan's syndrome, 38
Sensitization
  defined, 131
  vs. irritation, 13
Shoes, athletic, patch testing, 79
Skin cancer
  arsenic, inorganic, 94–95
  ionizing radiation, 95

Skin cancer (*contd.*)
  malignant melanoma, 95–96
  polycyclic hydrocarbons, 94
  ultraviolet light, 95
Specific occupations, allergen series for, 66–68
"Standard tray," for patch testing, 54–69
Systemic, defined, 131

T

Tape, patch testing, 44
Temperature, reaction to, 99
Temporal association, between exposure, and dermatitis onset, 114–115
Terminology, industrial hygiene, 118–123
Test application, patch testing, 44–46
Test system, patch testing, 44
Textile colors/finish series, patch testing, 67
Textile dye, patch testing, 77–78
Textile workers, patch testing, 77–78
Thioglycolates, irritant contact dermatitis, 7
Thiuram mix
  allergic contact dermatitis, 10
  patch testing, 60
Threshold limit value, defined, 119
Time frame, between exposure, and dermatitis onset, 114–115
Tinea manuum, diagnosis, 32
Toenail changes, 100
Topical medications, patch testing, 64–65
Traumatic irritant contact dermatitis, 17–18
Treatment
  allergic contact dermatitis, 108–109
  irritant contact dermatitis, 107–108
  occupational dermatitis, 104–111
    antibiotics, 106
    barrier cream, 105
    emollients, 106–107
    general principles, 104
    hand washing, 106
    protective gloves, 105–106
True test
  patch test, 44, 157

U

Ultraviolet light, skin cancer, 95
Unmasking, defined, 131
Unscheduled injury, defined, 131–132

V

Vesicobullous disease, diagnosis, 37
Virus infection, 96

W

Water, irritant contact dermatitis, 5
Wool alcohol, patch testing, 65
Workers' compensation board, 129–140
  sample letters, 133–139
Workup, occupationally related disorder, possible, 114

X

Xerotic eczema, diagnosis, 35